When Your Spouse Has a Stroke

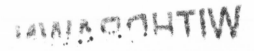

A Johns Hopkins Press Health Book

When Your Spouse Has a Stroke

*Caring for Your Partner, Yourself,
and Your Relationship*

Sara Palmer, Ph.D., and Jeffrey B. Palmer, M.D.

The Johns Hopkins University Press
Baltimore

Note to the Reader. This book is not meant to substitute for medical care of people with stroke, and treatment should not be based solely on its contents. Instead, treatment must be developed in a dialogue between the individual and his or her physician. Our book has been written to help with that dialogue.

© 2011 Sara Palmer, Ph.D., and Jeffrey B. Palmer, M.D.
All rights reserved. Published 2011
Printed in the United States of America on acid-free paper
9   8   7   6   5   4   3   2   1

The Johns Hopkins University Press
2715 North Charles Street
Baltimore, Maryland 21218-4363
www.press.jhu.edu

Library of Congress Cataloging-in-Publication Data
Palmer, Sara.
   When your spouse has a stroke : caring for your partner, yourself, and your relationship / Sara Palmer, and Jeffrey B. Palmer.
      p. cm. — (A Johns Hopkins Press health book)
   Includes bibliographical references and index.
   ISBN-13: 978-0-8018-9886-0 (hardcover : alk. paper)
   ISBN-10: 0-8018-9886-2 (hardcover : alk. paper)
   ISBN-13: 978-0-8018-9887-7 (pbk. : alk. paper)
   ISBN-10: 0-8018-9887-0 (pbk. : alk. paper)
   1. Cerebrovascular disease—Popular works. 2. Cerebrovascular disease—Patients—Family relationships—Popular works. 3. Cerebrovascular disease—Patients—Rehabilitation—Popular works. 4. Caregivers—Popular works. I. Palmer, Jeffrey B. II. Title.
   RC388.5.P34 2011
   616.8′1—dc22   2010025296

A catalog record for this book is available from the British Library.

Special discounts are available for bulk purchases of this book. For more information, please contact Special Sales at 410-516-6936 or specialsales@press.jhu.edu.

The Johns Hopkins University Press uses environmentally friendly book materials, including recycled text paper that is composed of at least 30 percent post-consumer waste, whenever possible. All of our book papers are acid-free, and our jackets and covers are printed on paper with recycled content.

For our parents,
Irving Sarnoff and Barbara and Walter Palmer

And in loving memory of
Suzanne Sarnoff

Contents

Acknowledgments

We are thankful to the many stroke survivors and their caregiver partners and spouses whom we have cared for over the years for allowing us to play a part in their physical and emotional recovery after stroke. Their struggles and triumphs were a major source of inspiration for this book.

Our work on caregiving was made possible by the generosity of many couples who volunteered to be interviewed about the effects of stroke on their marriage. They gave freely of their precious time and spoke openly about their experiences, good and bad. Their stories of problems and solutions, agreements and compromises, frustrations and satisfactions, sadness and humor, anger and love, fear and hope form the backbone of this book.

We appreciate the assistance of the speech language pathologists, social workers, and occupational therapists who invited us to share preliminary ideas for the book at stroke clubs and support groups, where we obtained indispensable feedback from stroke survivors and caregivers.

We thank our colleagues in the Johns Hopkins University Department of Physical Medicine and Rehabilitation, the Good Samaritan Hospital of Maryland, and the Johns Hopkins Bloomberg School of Public Health for enriching our knowledge and understanding of stroke and caregiving, for providing essential information on caregiver resources, and for their encouragement and interest in this book.

Jacqueline Wehmueller, our editor at the Johns Hopkins University Press, enriched the quality of the book with her invaluable insights and suggestions. Lois R. Crum's copyediting improved the clarity of the final manuscript.

Finally, we could not have written this book without a steady supply of support from our families and many wonderful friends. We thank them all for their love and patience.

When Your Spouse Has a Stroke

Setting the Stage for Life after Stroke

Stroke Happens to Both of You

Stroke happens—suddenly, unpredictably, and more frequently than you might think. Every year in the United States alone, about 795,000 people have a stroke, and there are currently about 6 million stroke survivors living in this country. If you are reading this book, you are most likely the spouse* of a stroke survivor; when stroke happened to your partner, it really happened to both of you. The stroke affects your life, immediately and over the long term, as well as your partner's life. If your spouse's stroke was recent, you know that a stroke can turn your own world upside down in an instant. And if you've had some time to adjust, you know that the effects of your spouse's stroke on your emotional health and your relationship can be far-reaching.

When your spouse has a stroke, you feel its shock waves. Stroke is often terrifying, and you may feel unprepared to cope with its immediate effects or its long-term consequences. But despite your lack of experience or preparation, you are likely to be the first one called upon to respond, make decisions, and provide for your spouse's care. You will probably assume the role of primary caregiver and begin a course of "on-the-job training."

If you are like most couples, the stroke will significantly affect your marriage; and it will affect your own physical and emotional health as

*In this book we use the terms *wife*, *husband*, and *spouse*. Our intention is for these terms to include anyone who is in a committed, long-term, intimate relationship.

well as your spouse's. Whether you are young or old, married for a few years or for decades, your spouse's stroke can be the biggest challenge of your married life. Like many other loving and committed spouses, you will no doubt do your best to help your spouse recover, no matter what difficulties you encounter. Our goal is to make your job easier, by helping you to anticipate problems that you and your spouse may encounter in the course of recovery from stroke and by offering ideas and resources to help you find solutions.

How This Book Can Help

One of us (Sara) is a rehabilitation psychologist and the other (Jeffrey) is a physiatrist (a doctor specializing in physical medicine and rehabilitation). In our professional lives, we have cared for stroke survivors and their spouses for more than 25 years. During this time, changes in the health care delivery system have resulted in shorter stays for stroke survivors in both the acute hospital and the inpatient rehabilitation unit. The nursing staffs of many hospitals struggle to keep up with basic patient care, and social workers are often preoccupied with other tasks as they make arrangements for the person's care after leaving the hospital and communicate with insurance companies to ensure patient benefits. There is little opportunity to educate the spouse about her role as caregiver, or even to provide adequate information on what to expect in terms of recovery from the stroke. Spouses may arrive home without a clear sense of what to do and with little preparation for problems they will encounter as caregivers.

There are, fortunately, many sources of general information about stroke and, increasingly, about caregiving and the needs of caregivers. And support for caregivers is available through several national stroke societies, organizations for caregivers, and many stroke rehabilitation hospitals. There are also books about family caregivers, addressed to a mixed audience of spouses, adult children, and other relatives who care for individuals with a variety of medical problems and disabilities. However, there appears to be little information available regarding the effects of stroke on *marriage* or the unique ways that caregiving affects spouses. Aside from individual memoirs, we could not find a book specifically addressing *spouse caregivers of stroke survivors,* nor any dealing with one of the critical issues for this group—how to maintain, improve, or rebuild a satisfying marriage after a stroke.

This book does just that, by discussing and offering solutions for many of the relationship problems you will experience after your spouse's stroke. We believe, based on our clinical experience, that knowing what to expect is an essential ingredient in coping effectively with problems that arise after stroke. Learning about a range of problems that other couples have confronted, and how they have solved them, can help you put your own experience in perspective. It will help you anticipate problems in your own marriage and develop your own solutions. This book will also prepare you for managing caregiving in a way that balances the difficult task of providing the best care for your spouse with the equally important task of taking care of *yourself.*

The information and advice we offer are based on our extensive experience caring for stroke survivors and their spouses at Johns Hopkins School of Medicine; our own research on stroke and caregiving, and that of others; feedback from participants in stroke clubs and support groups; and in-depth interviews of people living with stroke and their spouse caregivers. The people we interviewed were volunteers living in the community months or years after stroke.* Their candid and open discussions of their relationships were invaluable in preparing this book, and you will "meet" them in vignettes throughout the book, illustrating a variety of problems and solutions and sharing their insights. This book will provide you with information and guidance that will help you become a better caregiver for your spouse, take better care of your own needs as an individual, and continue to experience a satisfying marriage after your spouse's stroke.

You will need a basic knowledge of stroke to understand what has happened to your spouse and provide the best care. In the next few pages, we explain these stroke basics—what a stroke is, stroke types, and common consequences. Then we take a brief look at the important roles spouse caregivers play at home, as partners in the recovery of their husbands and wives, as well as in society, as health care partners

---

*In all cases, the identities of patients and interviewees have been disguised to protect their privacy and they have been given pseudonyms. Some of the stories in the book are composites based on multiple interviewees and clinical cases.

whose service makes a valuable social and economic contribution. Finally, we give you an overview of the coming chapters and how they can guide you to success as a caregiver when your spouse has had a stroke.

What Exactly *Is* a Stroke?

We had been planning to go away that evening for a week at an elderhostel. Everything had been going so well for us. My husband was in good health and very successful. He was semiretired and we were enjoying our free time together. But when I came home from the store to get ready, I found him collapsed on the basement floor. He wasn't able to talk and he couldn't move his right side. He couldn't stand up. I called 911 and they flew him to the hospital. I was so scared, I was numb. I didn't understand what was happening to him.—Carla, wife and caregiver

A stroke is a sudden loss of function of the brain caused by the death of brain cells. The brain is composed of tiny nerve cells called *neurons* that function like tiny computers with complex interconnections. They require a constant supply of blood to bring them essential nutrients and oxygen and carry away poisonous waste products. *Without an adequate supply of blood, brain cells rapidly lose function and die; this is basically what a stroke is.*

A stroke is often called a *cerebrovascular accident* (or *CVA*), the prefix "cerebro-" having to do with the brain, "vascular" referring to blood vessels, and "accident" meaning a sudden catastrophic event; or a *cerebral infarction,* meaning death of brain matter. Sometimes a stroke is referred to as a "brain attack," because the mechanism of stroke is similar to that of a heart attack.

A stroke can be the end result of a medical condition developing over many years, or it can be an unexpected event in an otherwise healthy person. Strokes occur more often in older people but can happen at any age. Unlike the well-known symptoms of a heart attack, the signs and symptoms of a stroke are not familiar to most people, and many are unsure what to do if they suspect that someone is having a stroke. Because its symptoms are harder to recognize, people often do not seek medical attention for many hours after the onset of a stroke. But a stroke is a medical emergency, and the affected person should be taken to a hospital immediately, preferably by a trained emergency medical crew, because actions taken in the first minutes or hours can lead to a dramatically higher survival rate and a better long-term outcome.

A stroke usually causes a sudden, dramatic change, such as loss of consciousness, paralysis, or the inability to speak and understand language, but sometimes these symptoms develop over a period of several hours.

> Life was beautiful. We were spending Thanksgiving weekend with our grandchildren. That Sunday my husband came in from raking the leaves, and he was so tired. He had a headache and I thought maybe he should call the doctor, but he didn't want to. He felt bad the rest of the day, and then after dinner, he came into the kitchen and he was swaying like he was going to fall. He kept saying "I don't know what's going on . . ." and then his words got all garbled. Then I thought it must be a stroke, and I called 911.—Josie, wife and caregiver

Different Types of Stroke

The outcome of stroke varies greatly, depending on the type of stroke, which brain area is affected, the size of the damaged area, how quickly treatment is given, what type of rehabilitation is available, and many other factors. There are two main types of stroke, which differ in their underlying causes as well as their effect on the brain. Doctors need to quickly determine which type of stroke a person has had, so measures can be taken to reduce the brain damage. Appropriate treatment is dramatically different for the two main types, ischemic and hemorrhagic. The type of stroke is usually best determined by images of the brain made with a CT (computerized tomography) scan or MRI (magnetic resonance imaging), so going to the hospital *immediately* is terribly important.

Ischemic Stroke

The most common type of stroke, *ischemic* stroke, is caused by obstruction of blood vessels to the brain, resulting in a critical loss of blood supply (ischemia) to an area of the brain. Ischemic strokes can be caused by any process that blocks the blood supply to the brain. One common subtype is known as *thrombotic* or *occlusive* stroke. In this disorder, a large blood vessel becomes narrower over a period of years because of atherosclerosis (hardening of the arteries). This is the same process that causes a heart attack, but in the case of stroke, it happens in the blood vessels going to the brain. A stroke results when the blood vessel is so narrow that the blood cannot flow.

An occlusive stroke affects an area on only one side of the brain, although that area can be large. This type of stroke can sometimes be treated with a "clot-busting" drug such as tissue plasminogen activator (tPA), which provides the best chance for reversing brain damage after an occlusive stroke. But there is a catch: the tPA must be given within three hours of the onset of the stroke. Giving tPA more than three hours after the stroke is not only useless; it is downright dangerous, because it can cause bleeding in the brain, a serious complication (see "Hemorrhagic Stroke," opposite). Because it takes some time to do a neurological examination and conduct the medical tests that are necessary before tPA can be given safely, a person experiencing stroke symptoms has an urgent problem and must get to the hospital as quickly as possible.

A second type of ischemic stroke is a *lacunar* stroke. This involves much smaller blood vessels of the brain than thrombotic stroke does. Disease in these smaller vessels is usually caused by many years of high blood pressure. As in thrombotic stroke, the blood vessels get narrower and narrower over the years, and when a vessel is too narrow for blood to flow through it, brain cells can die, causing a stroke. Because it involves tiny blood vessels, a lacunar stroke usually affects a small part of the brain, so it can be very mild; sometimes the person affected is not even aware of having a stroke. However, the narrowing of many small blood vessels can cause a series of lacunar strokes that occur over years. The cumulative effect of numerous small lacunar strokes can be severe.

The third major type of ischemic stroke is an *embolic* stroke. This type occurs when a blood clot or other solid matter (called an *embolus*) gets into the bloodstream and travels to the brain. If the embolus reaches a narrow blood vessel, it can get stuck there and block the flow of blood, causing a stroke. The size and location of the stroke depends on the size and location of the blood vessels that are blocked; blockage of larger vessels can result in a larger stroke. Sometimes multiple small blood clots enter the bloodstream and reach different parts of the brain at the same time. In that case, distant parts of the brain can be damaged simultaneously, causing complex patterns of stroke involving both sides of the brain.

The heart is the most common source for an embolus that travels to the brain. Blood clots or other foreign matter can accumulate in the heart and sometimes break apart there; then pieces can travel through the blood stream to the brain, where they can become lodged in a blood vessel and obstruct blood flow. This may happen in people who have an abnormal heart rhythm or disease of the heart valves.

Hemorrhagic Stroke

The second major category of stroke, *hemorrhagic* stroke, is caused by bleeding inside the head. Most often, the bleeding is inside the brain itself; this is called *intracerebral* hemorrhage ("intra-" means inside, and "cerebral" refers to the brain) and is usually caused by years of high blood pressure, especially if the high blood pressure has not been effectively treated. (Treatment of high blood pressure commonly involves salt restriction, exercise, and medication.) Intracerebral hemorrhages vary greatly in size. The bleeding can cause damage to the brain tissue directly around it or to parts of the brain that are far removed from it (by causing high pressure inside the brain). It is crucial to recognize when a stroke is caused by hemorrhage, rather than ischemia; while treatment of an ischemic stroke can require clot-busters or blood thinners, giving these drugs to a person immediately after a hemorrhagic stroke can cause more bleeding, a larger stroke, or even death.

Less commonly, there is bleeding between the skull and the *dura mater*, the tough membrane that covers the brain. This is called an *epidural* hemorrhage and usually occurs with a significant head injury. In contrast, a *subdural* hemorrhage can be caused by a minor blow to the head or can occur in the absence of any trauma. A subdural hemorrhage is bleeding *inside* the dura mater, where the blood vessels are more delicate, and can occur several days after the minor injury that caused it. A CT or an MRI scan is essential to make an accurate diagnosis.

Deeper inside the skull is the *arachnoid* membrane. Bleeding under this membrane is called a *subarachnoid* hemorrhage and is caused by the rupture of abnormal blood vessels, such as an *aneurysm* (abnormal enlargement of vessels) or an *arteriovenous malformation (AVM),* an abnormality of blood vessels that connect an artery to a vein. Any hemorrhage in or around the brain can cause a severe stroke, and surgery is sometimes necessary to stop the bleeding and remove the accumulated blood.

Other Types of Stroke

There are many other uncommon kinds of stroke, far too numerous to mention; an exhaustive discussion is beyond the scope of this book. For more detailed information on the full variety of stroke causes, symptoms, and consequences that might match your spouse's more closely, we refer you to the excellent books and national organizations dedicated to stroke that are listed in Resources at the end of this book. Your physician can also provide additional information about the cause of your spouse's stroke and can suggest steps you and your spouse can take to prevent another stroke (stroke prevention is discussed further in chapter 6). What all strokes have in common is the death of brain cells, caused by disease of the brain's blood vessels and resulting in either disrupted blood flow or bleeding.

Consequences of Stroke

A stroke can have many possible consequences because it can affect any part of the brain, and various parts of the brain control various specific functions. For example, language is primarily controlled by the left side of the brain. Voluntary movements of the arms and legs are primarily controlled by the opposite side of the brain (for example, the left side of the body is controlled by the right side of the brain). Control of alertness relies on a large area of the brain, so damage in many different parts of the brain can lead to lethargy, fatigue, sleepiness, or even coma. A very small stroke can have minimal effects if it is in an area of the brain that does not control any critical brain functions. But a very small stroke in the *brain stem,* an area that controls critical functions such as breathing and swallowing, can have significant effects on basic life functions.

There are far more possible consequences of a stroke than we can cover in this book, and they can occur either alone or in combination. We will discuss several common conditions that result from stroke.

Hemiplegia

One of the most common disabling effects of stroke is weakness or paralysis. In most cases, it affects just one side of the body and is known as *hemiplegia* (paralysis) or *hemiparesis* (weakness). The weakness ranges from total paralysis of the entire side, including the face, tongue, and trunk muscles on that side, to mild weakness of one limb; it depends on the location and size of the stroke. Hemiplegia can also produce changes in muscle tone. If the muscle tone of an arm or a leg is greatly increased, the limb may become very stiff and difficult to move. In some cases, strength is normal but movement is extremely limited because of a condition called spasticity, one form of muscle tone that is commonly increased after stroke. Strength and muscle tone often change over time following a stroke, and they frequently improve with therapy.

Incoordination

Another kind of problem with movement after a stroke is loss of coordination. This can occur when the control of movement is not well organized by the brain; it results in clumsy or ineffective movement. A common type of incoordination, called *ataxia*, may affect movements of the limbs or the trunk, ranging from mild incoordination, in which a movement looks clumsy but is effective (say, in picking up a pencil), to a severe condition that makes it impossible to walk or perform the simplest kinds of voluntary movement. Ataxia commonly results from damage to a specialized area on the back of the brain called the *cerebellum*, but it can also be caused by damage to other parts of the brain.

Loss of Sensation

A stroke can cause partial or total loss of feeling (sensation) in a part of the body or on one side of the body. For example, one can lose the ability to sense heat and cold on one side or have diminished sensitivity to painful stimulation on the face, an arm, or a leg. In some cases, sensation is present but abnormal; for example, a gentle touch might produce a tingling or burning sensation. A stroke can also affect vision. Sometimes a person loses vision on only one side but it involves both eyes. If that happens, the person cannot see things on the left side using either the right eye or the left eye. This is called *hemianopia*. Rarely, a stroke may involve one of the optic nerves, the nerve that carries visual information from one eye to the brain, causing blindness in that eye and having no effect on the other eye.

Pain

Many individuals have pain after a stroke. Most pain after stroke is related to joints, tendons, and muscles or related to damaged brain centers.

Weakness and abnormal muscle tone resulting from a stroke cause abnormal stresses and strains on the muscles and joints, especially in the shoulders, hands, hips, knees, and ankles. These pains can be prevented by careful attention to posture and positioning and can be treated much as they would be in an able-bodied person (with heat, cold, slings, splints, or physical therapy). In other cases, the pain may be a direct result of damage to brain centers that control pain sensation or nerve cells that carry pain signals from one area of the brain to another. This pain is commonly called *central* pain or *neurogenic* pain, and it may not respond to ordinary painkillers such as Tylenol, Advil, or even opiates such as OxyContin. If the pain is severe, it can be treated with special medications that alter the function of brain cells in these pain centers. Among the drugs that are used are some that were developed to treat other conditions, such as antidepressants and medications for epileptic seizures.

Difficulty Swallowing

About half of the people who have a stroke experience difficulty swallowing, known as *dysphagia*. In some cases, food or drink can "go down the wrong pipe" during swallowing and cause coughing and choking. When food goes into the windpipe, an event called *aspiration,* it can cause a potentially very serious complication: aspiration pneumonia, a common cause of death in the first few days after a stroke. Nowadays, a person who has had a stroke receives a screening test for dysphagia on the day of the stroke and is frequently checked for signs of pneumonia such as fever or cough.

Good medical techniques have reduced the risk of pneumonia caused by dysphagia and greatly improved the chance of surviving a stroke. A person who has experienced a stroke and has difficulty swallowing is evaluated by a speech language pathologist and undergoes analysis of his swallowing by fluoroscopy, a type of video x-ray that shows aspiration and other abnormalities and permits the clinicians to test techniques for preventing aspiration. These techniques can include diet modifications, special ways of breathing, and different ways of swallowing, such as with changes in posture, head position, or timing. For the majority of people with dysphagia after a stroke, their swallowing improves and they eventually return to a normal diet. But for some, swallowing creates such high risk of pneumonia that it is best to avoid it altogether (at least temporarily) and instead to take food and drink through a tube that passes directly into the stomach.

Bladder and Bowel Problems

Many people lose the ability to control their urine after a stroke. This is called incontinence of bladder. For most people with stroke, this incontinence is a temporary condition related to loss of alertness and confusion in the first few days after a stroke. During this time, one way to prevent "accidents" is to insert a catheter (either into the bladder or, for men, attached to a condom that is placed on the penis). Adult diapers are preferable in some cases, but the advantage of a catheter is that it makes it easy for the medical staff to measure the urine and make sure the person's fluid output and input are balanced. Some people become dehydrated because they don't drink enough fluids after a stroke, and dehydration can be detected and treated if urine output is monitored carefully.

For some people, a stroke affects the areas of the brain that normally control the bladder and urinary function, resulting in continuing incontinence. Many of these people are able to regain control of urination though a bladder training program that involves behavioral treatment and may include medication.

Older men often have difficulty urinating because of benign enlargement of the prostate, even if they are otherwise healthy. A man's prostate enlargement is not affected by a stroke, but his difficulty with urination is likely to get worse because of weakness or incoordination of bladder muscles. The treatment is basically the same as for other people with incontinence caused by stroke, except that for men with prostate enlargement, it is especially important to make sure they can empty their bladders by urination. Otherwise, a range of treatments are available, including catheters, medications, bladder training, and in severe cases, surgery.

Constipation is typical after a stroke and may result simply from taking in less food and being less mobile. It is usually treated by taking stool softeners and laxatives. Some people become incontinent of bowel and have stool "accidents," but this problem usually improves with a bowel training program. Nurses and doctors who specialize in rehabilitation are knowledgeable about bowel and bladder problems and how to treat them.

Speech and Language Effects

A stroke often causes *aphasia*, or an interference with the stroke survivor's ability to express ideas through words (either spoken or written) or to understand language by listening or reading. There are several types of aphasia, ranging from minimal to very severe. When aphasia is most severe, the person cannot understand any spoken or written words or use words to express himself at all. In that event, it may be possible to communicate to some extent with gestures, symbols, and facial expressions. Aphasia usually results from damage to the left side of the brain, so many people with aphasia also have right hemiparesis, weakness on their right side.

Another type of communication impairment is *dysarthria*, which involves difficulty producing speech because of weakness or incoordination of the lips, tongue, and throat muscles but does not affect language function as controlled by the brain. The stroke survivor's speech may be slurred or even unintelligible, but she knows exactly what she wants to say, has no trouble finding the right words, and has no difficulty with reading, writing, or comprehending speech. If the vocal cords are weak or not coordinated, her speech will sound hoarse, a condition called *dysphonia*. A speech therapist can provide treatment for these conditions.

Cognitive Deficits

A stroke can alter a person's thinking, memory, and other cognitive processes. It often affects alertness, which is fundamental to cognitive function. In the early stages of recovery, the stroke survivor can be very sleepy and difficult to wake up. His level of alertness can wax and wane for the first few days after a stroke, and minor changes are to be expected. A sudden severe loss of consciousness, however, can indicate another stroke, a seizure, or an infection. A stroke commonly interferes with a person's attention span and ability to concentrate, making him easily distracted. It can also impair judgment, making it difficult for him to make sound decisions about his care and safety, personal relationships, finances, or life plans.

A particularly difficult set of problems is known as unawareness or inattention syndromes. These effects occur mostly in strokes affecting the right side of the brain but can occur with a stroke in some other location. The two common types are unawareness of illness and condition (technically called *anosognosia*) and spatial inattention. With unawareness of illness, a person may have difficulty recognizing that she has had a stroke or that she has physical impairments. For example, with this condition a person may deny having had a stroke or may be unable to recognize that part of her body is paralyzed or weak. It is important to emphasize that unawareness of illness in a person recovering from stroke is a direct result of damage to the brain and does not reflect stubbornness or weakness of will. This neurological unawareness of illness is sometimes, confusingly, called "physiological denial" of illness. But it is entirely different from the psychological defense mechanism known as "denial," in which a person denies that he is having a strong emotional response to a life event.

Spatial inattention refers to lack of awareness or attention to a part of space. This occurs most often after a right-brain stroke and usually involves unawareness of the left side of space; it is often called left-neglect. A person with visual inattention may be unable to pay attention to people or things on the left, or even to look to the left, and may behave as though she is blind on the left although her sense of vision is normal. A person with left spatial inattention may be unable to recognize or pay attention to anything on his left side. Spatial inattention can affect all spatial senses, perceptions, and thoughts related to "leftness." For example, a person can fail to notice food on the left side of a plate and may repeatedly walk into barriers located on the left, creating a risk of bodily harm. In severe cases, the person might not be able to find or even to recognize his left arm or leg as a part of his body.

Disturbances of Mood and Emotion

People recovering from a stroke can have difficulty controlling their emotions. There may be inappropriate outbursts at some times and an apparent lack of emotional response at other times. Outward expressions of emotion, such as crying, may not reflect the person's experience of sadness or distress but instead can result from any kind of emotional arousal. This condition is called *emotional lability*.

About half of people recovering from strokes develop a poststroke depressive disorder. This is a specific psychiatric disorder that is caused, in part, by damage to the brain. Highly effective, relatively inexpensive treatments are available, including medications and psychotherapy. Common symptoms of depressive disorder experienced by people with stroke include insomnia, loss of appetite, irritability, and loss of interest in activities that were previously pleasurable. Often the depressed person does not say she feels sad or depressed, even though she has other severe symptoms of depression. Recognizing and treating depression is extraordinarily important because it can deeply affect a person's physical functioning, relationships, and recovery from stroke, and it can move a person to suicide.

The term for all of these conditions in which brain damage caused by a stroke causes changes in emotions, perceptions, and behavior is *neurobehavioral syndromes*.

Diminished Mobility and Self-Care Skills

People recovering from a stroke can find it very difficult to walk or propel a wheelchair (mobility) and may have diminished self-care skills (commonly called *activities of daily living* or *ADLs*). Restoring these skills is a major focus of rehabilitation and the primary goal of physical and occupational therapy. Therapists conduct two kinds of treatments. One kind is activity geared toward recovering strength, sensation, and control of the body. Another kind attempts to improve the person's ability to perform functional activities such as moving between different sitting surfaces, walking, self-feeding, dressing, bathing, and personal hygiene. Even if recovery is limited, learning new ways to move about and to care for oneself can make the difference between returning home to live with one's spouse and needing constant care in a nursing home.

The Course of Illness and the Prognosis for Recovery

The course of illness refers to the time it takes to recover and how the severity of illness changes over time. A stroke usually (not always) comes on suddenly, producing a rapid and dramatic loss of function over a short time. The affected person may be paralyzed, confused, or even unresponsive. The person's neurological function may actually worsen over the first few days because of swelling of the brain, which is common after a large stroke, but then begin to improve. The pattern of sudden loss of function followed by gradual improvement is typical of stroke recovery. *The good news is that, however severely a person is affected in the initial days after a stroke, almost every stroke survivor experiences gradual, significant improvement.* Sadly, a small number of people do very poorly and die in the first few days after a stroke. But of those who survive this critical period, few die from later complications of stroke. If you are reading this book, your spouse has probably survived and is in the stage of gradually improving, but you may be uncertain how much recovery to expect.

We can state that most people improve after a stroke, but we can't be much more precise, because different stroke survivors vary so much in both rate and extent of recovery. It is impossible to predict with certainty how quickly or slowly a given person will recover. Some people improve dramatically in a few weeks, while others improve very slowly over many years. In general, recovery gets slower as time passes, but it is very hard to know when a person's recovery has actually stopped. Some people will have such superb recovery that it is impossible to tell that they ever had a stroke; others will be left with some loss of physical or cognitive function.

Research on stem cell therapy shows promise for future improvements in recovery from a stroke. Most cells in the human body have a specific form and function that is unique to their particular role; for example, nerve cells (neurons) have a cell body and a very long, thin arm that can carry nerve signals to distant cells. But a stem cell does not have these unique features. It is a sort of undifferentiated or "generic" cell that can develop into a specialized cell, such as a neuron. The idea of stem cell therapy is that if stem cells are implanted in an area of the brain that has been damaged by a stroke, perhaps those stem cells can be turned into neurons that will make connections with the surrounding healthy brain neurons and reproduce the brain functions that were lost in the stroke.

At this time, we have the ability to implant stem cells, but we have only limited ability to program the stem cells to become brain neurons and connect themselves to the healthy neurons in the right way to undo a stroke's damage. Recent studies have shown encouraging results in animals with experimental stroke, and early clinical trials with human subjects are now in progress (though not yet in the United States). There is good reason to hope that these trials will be successful and that stem cell implants will one day play an important role in stroke recovery.

Rehabilitation of Stroke Survivors

Rehabilitation is crucial in enhancing recovery from a stroke, preventing complications, and ensuring that the person will regain as much normal function as possible. You might think it would make sense to put off rehabilitation until your spouse has had a chance to rest and recover strength and can fully understand what has happened. But that is absolutely incorrect. Rehabilitation needs to start immediately after a stroke; the earlier rehabilitation begins, the greater the chance of full recovery. However, if your spouse did not have early rehabilitation, there are some physical and other rehabilitation therapies that can be effective in improving function at a later point, even years after a stroke. It has been learned that modern techniques of rehabilitation can actually improve nerve connections in the brain as well as the ability to perform activities like walking and dressing.

For centuries, scientists believed that the adult brain was organized so that each area of the brain controlled only a specific set of functions, which were unchangeable. It was also thought that if an area of the brain was damaged, the function it performed (for example, language) would be lost permanently. But recent studies have shown that the brain can adapt to damage (as in a stroke) by changing its structure and functions through a process known as *plasticity*. This means that if one area of the brain is damaged, other areas, including the opposite side of the brain, can sometimes take over the function of the damaged area. These alterations in function can be demonstrated graphically with new noninvasive methods (such as functional MRI, also called fMRI) that can measure brain activity during behaviors such as moving the limbs, reading, or remembering.

Several new techniques for rehabilitation are showing promise for improving function by encouraging brain plasticity, even in people who have not been helped by traditional therapy. Constraint-induced therapy (CIT) is a new treatment for arm weakness after a stroke. CIT forces the person to use his affected (weak) arm by physically restraining use of his unaffected (strong) arm. The weak arm goes through intensive exercise while the unaffected arm is held in a sling. This seems to encourage the brain to adapt, improving the weak arm's strength and coordination.

Another new technique is functional electrical stimulation (FES), which directly stimulates nerves in the patient's affected limbs, forcing the muscles to contract and thus strengthening paralyzed muscles. If the stimulation is timed correctly, it can substitute for the damaged brain, making various muscles contract in the correct sequence for walking or other activities. FES can potentially promote recovery of movement in weak or paralyzed muscles, although its ability to bring about brain recovery is controversial.

A more recent development in rehabilitation research uses low-intensity electrical stimulation of the brain to encourage recovery after a stroke. The few preliminary studies that have been published seem to show that certain kinds of electrical stimulation applied to the scalp can enhance the function of the brain. It is too early to say whether this approach will help people regain lost abilities after a stroke. But just maybe, in the not-too-distant future, people recovering from stroke will wear battery packs that power electrical brain stimulation devices. What a change that would be!

Rehabilitation professionals, including doctors, nurses, therapists, psychologists, and social workers, can help you learn more about your spouse's particular impairments and how you can foster her recovery, improve your communication with her, and get additional help you may need with caregiving.

Caregiver Spouses: Partners in Stroke Recovery

The great majority of stroke survivors, whether or not they have some lasting impairment, can return to community living and resume active, fulfilling lives. Even when the physical, emotional, and financial costs of caregiving are particularly high, most people consider care at home to be the best alternative. Spouses make this possible for many stroke survivors—those who are married have a higher likelihood of receiving care at home than those who are single or widowed. And having a spouse is linked to better recovery of the stroke survivor's mobility and self-care. As a spouse caregiver, you provide not only physical care but essential emotional support. A good marriage plays a fundamental role in enhancing your spouse's inner strength, boosting his mood, motivating him to be more active, preventing stroke-related complications, and promoting the most rapid and complete recovery. Your spouse will benefit not only from receiving your care and support, but also from having opportunities to reengage as fully as possible in his role as a loving spouse and helpmate in your marriage and family life.

Research on couples after a stroke suggests that there is a reciprocal relationship between a stroke survivor and her spouse in which the function of each affects the other. If you have a well-functioning and emotionally supportive marriage, your spouse is likely to fare better both emotionally and in recovery of her physical and social functions. However, a stroke can create significant stress and challenges for a couple, making it difficult, even for couples who functioned well before the stroke, to maintain an emotionally supportive and close relationship. A stroke can cause the breakdown of a couple's usual coping mechanisms, leading to an increase in conflict and possibly depression or other emotional difficulties for the caregiving spouse. If you are depressed, anxious, or burned out, it is harder to give emotional support to your stroke-survivor spouse. Similarly, marital tensions and dissatisfaction may lead to greater distance between you and your spouse, resulting in fewer opportunities to support his recovery. Stroke survivors whose spouses are depressed, or whose relationships are strained and unfulfilling following the stroke, are more likely to become depressed themselves and may have worse health. Your spouse's best recovery depends in part on your own physical and mental health and the smooth functioning of your marriage. This means that finding ways to support and care for *yourself,* and to maintain a satisfying marriage, will help you in your mission to provide the best care possible for your spouse over the long haul.

Caregivers in Society

Family caregivers play an ever-increasing role in society, providing untold hours of care to aging relatives and family members with disabilities—care that would otherwise put a tremendous economic strain on the health care system. About 29 million family members care for an adult with a chronic illness or disability, and it is estimated that by 2050, the ranks of family caregivers will include about 37 million people. The expected increase is due in part to the recent shift of care responsibilities for people with disabilities from the medical center to the community, and it is due in part to the dramatic increase in the population of older adults—by 2030, there will be about 71 million Americans over 65 years of age (compared to fewer than 37 million in 2004).

More than half of family caregivers are also employed outside the home, and more than 60 percent are women. Many caregivers provide care to multiple family members, for example dependent children and elderly parents, in addition to caring for a spouse with a disability. Family caregivers receive no financial compensation, but they work hard and put in long hours.

In recent years, caregivers have been increasingly recognized both for the value of their service and for the strains they experience in fulfilling their multiple roles. Caregivers have become the focus of public health and psychosocial research aimed at finding ways to make their jobs easier and improve their quality of life. Because the special needs of caregivers are recognized by mental health professionals, the availability of support groups and therapy for caregivers has increased. Caregivers have become more involved in advocacy and public policy, and resources for caregivers have expanded dramatically in recent years. This trend is likely to continue in the years to come as the number of caregivers soars.

What You Will Find in This Book— and Where You'll Find It

The introduction explains how your spouse's stroke can affect you and your relationship. Common problems that may occur include emotional stress and feelings of loss, role changes, depression, social isolation, and changes in sexuality. You as the caregiver may experience physical strain, difficulty meeting your own health care needs, loss of leisure-time activities, and burnout. Some potential benefits that may arise as you tend to your spouse are increased emotional closeness, a shared sense of purpose, and the opportunity to change aspects of your marriage that were unsatisfactory prior to the stroke. You may find meaning and value in your caregiver role, and you may benefit from increased self-esteem and feelings of accomplishment.

In chapter 1 we focus on the role of social support in health and recovery after a stroke, how you can provide this support yourself, and how you can get support for your spouse from other sources. This chapter summarizes results of extensive research regarding the benefits of social support for health in general and specifically for mental and physical recovery after a stroke. We explain the various benefits of emotional support versus practical support for your spouse's recovery, as well as how a supportive marital relationship can reduce your spouse's risk for depression while increasing her activity.

Chapter 2 helps you balance the role of caregiver with your other marital, social, and work roles. This chapter looks at how you can avoid overprotecting your spouse, how you can include your spouse as a partner in solving problems and planning activities, how to create a more balanced or reciprocal relationship, and ideas for home-based hobbies and activities and social and leisure activities outside the home.

In chapter 3 we explore sexuality after a stroke, including the challenge of playing the double role of caregiver and romantic partner. This chapter addresses the psychological issues—such as fear of causing another stroke, difficulty talking about sex, and changes in body-image and self-esteem—that are the causes of most sexual problems after a stroke. We explain physiological difficulties with sexual function and treatments for these problems, and we discuss issues in sexual intimacy that relate to a spouse's significant cognitive impairment or inability to communicate.

In chapter 4 we highlight opportunities for *you*—the caregiver—to benefit from social and emotional support beyond what is available within your marital relationship. We discuss the value of both practical and emotional support for caregivers, including the importance of extended family, friendships, social activities, and stroke clubs or support groups. We also suggest paths you might follow in caring for yourself both physically and emotionally. In a section on caregiver advocacy, we discuss your rights as a caregiver, how to ensure that your needs are considered in care planning, and how to define your role independently of family or societal expectations.

In chapter 5 you can learn how to maintain a satisfying marriage after stroke, including how to help your marriage incorporate the effects of stroke-related disabilities and caregiving tasks and how to change relationship patterns that are not or never were working for you. The role of professional counseling to help with difficulties you may encounter in doing this on your own is also discussed. We identify roadblocks to restoring your marital relationship that can arise when your spouse has serious stroke-caused limitations in thinking, communication, or behavior.

In chapter 6, we begin with a discussion of what you and your spouse can do to help prevent another stroke and to maintain your physical health in general. As you and your spouse grow old together, both of you are almost certainly going to have some medical problems—that's just a fact of life. In this chapter, we help you think about planning for future health needs, including financial and legal matters, maintaining your relationship when your spouse needs care in a nursing home, and various end-of-life issues.

At the end of each chapter, we have listed some "Practical Tips."

This section is a summary of the advice and suggestions included in the chapter. You can refer to this list whenever you wish for a quick review of the material.

In the epilogue, which discusses the evolving role of caregivers in our society, we describe new intervention programs for caregivers and look at what caregivers are doing to help themselves and each other. Basically, we find an optimistic future for stroke survivors and caregivers. You and your spouse may want to share with other couples your own accumulated wisdom and insights on living as a couple with stroke, so we explain how you might go about doing that.

At the end of the book you will find a Resources section, which points you to sources on general stroke information and education, caregiver support, respite services, leisure activities, stroke clubs, and more.

INTRODUCTION

When Stroke Moves In

How Stroke Affects You and Your Marriage

In the prologue we focused, appropriately, on the person who has had a stroke. This person and this person's needs *must* come first, for a while. After the acute, critical period is past, however, it's time to make sure that you, the caregiving spouse, are appropriately cared for, too. In this introduction, we look at the ways your partner's stroke affects *you*, the caregiver, and how it affects your relationship.

You may have already experienced some of the challenges of coping with your spouse's stroke, becoming a caregiver, and trying to manage the impact of stroke on your marriage. When you care for *any* relative, the practical and physical demands are stressful, but caring for your *spouse* is complicated by the emotional effects of the stroke on your relationship.

Exactly how caregiving affects you and your marriage depends in large part on how much care your spouse requires, your attitudes about being a caregiver, the type of relationship you have with your spouse, the amount of support you have from others, and your preparation for caregiving. These pages can be part of your preparation. Each person's experience is unique, and you will not encounter all of the situations or have all of the feelings discussed. But by exposing you to the range of experiences you may have as a caregiver, this introduction can help you begin to anticipate problems, examine preventive strategies, and think about how to shape a better caregiving experience for *you*.

The Caregiver Experience

As the number of family caregivers has rapidly expanded in recent years, caregivers have come to be recognized as a distinct social group. They are partners with professional health care providers, and they make valuable contributions to the welfare of people with disabilities; but as a result of being caregivers, they are also vulnerable to particular social, physical, and mental health problems of their own. Much research has been devoted to better understanding the caregiving experience and to developing interventions to reduce caregivers' stress and improve their ability to cope.

Research on family caregivers shows that they are likely to experience "burden" or "strain," including anxiety and loneliness, and to feel overwhelmed by their responsibilities. Several changes in the lives of caregivers contribute to these problems. Many caregivers are stressed by changes in their social roles; in addition to their new caregiving tasks, they often take on other family responsibilities and chores that used to be done by the care recipient. Because caregivers often have less time to see their friends or pursue social activities, they may become socially isolated. They may be sleep-deprived and exhausted from the demands of providing 24–hour care, and their own physical health is likely to suffer. Limited opportunities for exercise, healthy meals, and relaxation add to caregiver stress. Spouse caregivers may be particularly distressed by their partner's increased dependency, or by cognitive and personality changes associated with neurological illnesses; disruptions in sexual and other aspects of their marital relationship are common for spouse caregivers. So it is no surprise that caregivers are more likely than others to experience clinical depression, social isolation, poor health, or burnout.

Of course, not all caregivers have all (or even any) of these problems. Many factors may make your experience very different from another caregiver's. Current research on the caregiver experience is focused on identifying specific caregiving problems associated with the care recipient's *diagnosis* (such as dementia, stroke, or paralysis), with particular points in *time* (right after diagnosis or after several years—or decades—of caregiving), and with the caregiver's *relationship* to the care recipient (spouse, parent, or sibling).

Researchers are also examining why some people adjust more easily to caregiving and experience less stress; caregivers who have better problem-solving skills and more social support and whose family life has included emotional closeness and good communication seem to have an easier time. Some caregivers even benefit psychologically: they may discover a new sense of purpose or develop greater self-esteem and confidence as a result of learning new tasks and taking on additional responsibilities. When things are going exceptionally well, caregivers may experience "uplifts"—special satisfactions or joys experienced in the course of caring for their spouse.

Much research on caregiver problems and interventions is based on caregivers of people with Alzheimer's disease (AD). But because stroke and AD are markedly different, the experience of caregivers is not the same. The course of AD is gradual, progressive, and degenerative. The gradual decline in function of the person with AD allows caregivers time to adapt, but as the disease progresses, the demands on the caregiver—and the likelihood of emotional and physical stress—increase dramatically. For people with stroke, the situation is quite different. Because stroke usually occurs suddenly and without warning, the functioning of the survivor is at its worst immediately after the stroke. There is almost always improvement over time, giving caregivers a chance to adapt and offering the potential to cope *better* with the passing years. Similarly, although stroke can take a toll on a marriage, the relationship can eventually "bounce back" as the stroke survivor regains function and learns how to accommodate to his remaining limitations.

Because stroke recovery is a "moving target," certain caregiver and marital problems may be more prominent at different points in time. A recent paper described five theoretical phases in stroke recovery that correspond with different challenges for stroke caregivers. This framework may help you better understand what to expect at each point in the process of recovery and what might be helpful to you during those phases.

The first phase starts with *diagnosis,* when your spouse has just had a stroke and is in the hospital. At this point, you probably are anxious about your spouse's survival and feel confused about her condition. You will benefit from information about stroke and from emotional support.

The second phase begins when your spouse's medical condition is *stabilized*, her abilities (for walking, speech, and so forth) are being evaluated, and she is showing some initial improvements. During this period, you probably feel relieved that your spouse has survived but worried about how her physical and cognitive impairments will affect your lives when she comes home. Waiting for the results of evaluations and a determination of your spouse's prognosis can be agonizing. You may benefit from counseling and support, from the hospital social worker or from friends and family.

During the third phase, *preparation,* your spouse is getting ready to leave the hospital, and you are wondering how you will take care of him at home. This can be a difficult time, because you need to learn how to care for him, arrange for home care and support services, and perhaps plan to go back to work after a leave of absence. You will benefit from referrals to community resources and supports, from ongoing emotional support, and from education to boost your confidence in your ability to provide care.

When your spouse comes home, the *implementation* phase begins. This is when the responsibility for your spouse's care shifts from the hospital to *you;* you will have to develop your own care routines, help your spouse adapt to the home environment, arrange transportation and appointments, manage meals and shopping, and so forth. During this time, caregivers often experience a loss of confidence in their abilities, as well as a lack of adequate community or social support. Awareness of the social and physical impact of caregiving begins to sink in, and you may feel sadness or loss. Telephone or Internet support programs, available through some stroke centers, can be helpful in this phase, when it is difficult to get out of the house.

The final phase, *adaptation,* starts when medical and rehabilitation therapies are complete; improvements in your spouse's function continue, but at a much slower pace. At this point, your needs will likely shift to include improving your social life, getting your spouse involved in activities outside the home, resuming your sexual relationship with your spouse, and exploring whether she can drive, do her normal work, or travel. You may experience more stress in juggling your multiple needs and responsibilities and will benefit from caregiver support groups and help from people who can give you a break from caregiving. Concerns about the future, your own health, and how to manage your own and your spouse's long-term-care needs may arise at this time.

All of these issues are explored in more detail in this introduction and in the rest of the book. We discuss how you can prevent and solve problems, become a more effective caregiver, take better care of yourself, and improve your relationship with your spouse. You will see that while stroke has the potential to create strain, frustration, and distance in your marriage, coping with the effects of your spouse's stroke can also be an opportunity to reset your priorities and goals. You may be able to strengthen your marriage as you and your spouse work together on the common problems you will face when stroke "moves in."

Stresses and Strains of Caregiving

Anxiety, Loss, and Grief

Georgia and Howie had been married for 10 years when Georgia had multiple embolic strokes, resulting from complications of an acute illness. Georgia had had several chronic conditions over the years, but she had been able to work and raise her daughter, Suzy, as a single mom. She married Howie when Suzy was in college. A devoted husband, Howie worked hard as manager of a supermarket, helped Georgia with housework, and accompanied her to doctors' appointments. They shared many common interests, including movies, cooking, entertaining family, walking in local parks, and attending church functions. They enjoyed an affectionate, easygoing relationship, a good sex life, and mutual support. Howie had become used to the ups and downs of Georgia's health, and on her "bad days" he was happy to spend quiet time with her at home. But when Georgia suddenly became so ill that he "almost lost her," Howie was devastated. Her strokes resulted in paralysis on her left side, slurred speech, and confusion in her thinking, and Howie knew that this would be the biggest challenge of their lives together so far.

After treatment in the Intensive Care Unit and a medical unit, Georgia spent two weeks in a rehabilitation hospital, where she learned to walk with a walker, dress and bathe herself with one hand, and speak more slowly to improve her pronunciation. When she came home, Howie took a leave from work to become her full-time caregiver. He had no difficulty assisting Georgia with homemaking tasks or helping her into the bathtub, but he was dismayed by Georgia's difficulty in organizing her thoughts and remembering what he told her. She had always been soft-spoken and had had a good sense of humor, but now there was something "off" about her personality. She seemed childish and passive, and she often giggled for no apparent reason. Howie worried that Georgia would never be quite herself again. While he continued to be affectionate toward her, he was hesitant to approach her sexually. For one thing, her apparent lack of interest in sex and her mental "fuzziness" were off-putting, and for another, he was afraid that sexual activity might cause her to have another stroke.

Howie also wasn't sure how much to push Georgia when she didn't feel like going to church or visiting their families. He didn't want to boss her around, but he was concerned that if he didn't take a firm stand, Georgia would be content to stay home all the time. Howie began to feel cut off from family and friends, and he was frustrated because he couldn't motivate Georgia. He missed his job but was afraid of leaving Georgia alone all day. Feelings of sadness and loneliness crept up on him over a few months, and Howie soon found himself with a "mild case of the blues."

Spouses are likely to feel anxious after a partner's stroke, especially when the stroke causes changes in behavior, thinking, or emotional expression, as in Georgia's case. When this occurs, you can feel alienated from your spouse, or experience him as being "a different person." Anxiety can be heightened by uncertainty about whether these changes in behavior will improve and by questions about how much control the stroke survivor has over his behavior. It will probably be helpful to discuss these behaviors with your spouse's doctor or rehabilitation professionals to learn whether these changes are the result of brain damage. Your reaction to your spouse's behavior may be different if you know that it is not the result of willfulness or changes in his feelings for you.

You may also be worried that your spouse might have another stroke, especially if the stroke was related to medical risk factors that persist, such as diabetes, high blood pressure, or smoking. There are about 200,000 cases of recurrent stroke each year in the United States. Fortunately, better management of health behaviors (diet, exercise, smoking cessation, treatment for depression, and so forth) after a stroke help reduce the risk of a second stroke. (Strategies for stroke prevention are addressed in detail in chapter 6.)

Loss and grief are also common responses to a spouse's stroke. Like Howie, you may experience feelings of loss because of your spouse's changes in personality, emotional expression, or cognitive ability, or your spouse may have aphasia, severely reducing your ability to communicate. These changes can have profound effects on all aspects of the marriage by limiting intimacy, companionship, and emotional support. You may grieve the loss of your partner's physical abilities, even if her thinking and personality are unaffected. If your spouse is no longer able to do the things you both used to enjoy or is physically unable to perform valuable tasks such as driving a car, caring for the children, or working, both of you may experience a period of sadness, and you may grieve for these lost abilities. If the stroke affects your spouse both physically and mentally, you may feel bereft of the emotional and practical support you used to enjoy.

Anger

Sometimes your frustration in relating to your spouse after his abilities have changed dramatically can spill over into anger.

> Rita knows that her husband, Paul, is unable to initiate many behaviors and that he is frequently uncooperative because of changes in his brain function after two strokes, and usually it doesn't bother her. But sometimes, she says, she feels "angry and discouraged. I get upset with him because he doesn't try, doesn't make the effort to walk," and it seems as if "he's causing his own problems."

Like Rita, even if you know your spouse can't always control his behavior, you may still feel angry or hold him responsible for the effects of his stroke—you're only human! But anger is a difficult emotion for many caregiving spouses to accept; they may feel guilty about getting angry at their spouse and try to squelch their feelings, rather than finding constructive ways to cope with them. One caregiver put it this way: "We've never had a fight where we yelled at each other . . . just a lot of cold wars!" While yelling at each other is not usually helpful, expressing your anger with "the silent treatment" or holding in your feelings until you "snap" can increase your emotional stress when caring for a spouse who has cognitive limitations or changes in personality. Rita has learned to cope with these feelings by expressing them to supportive friends, which has helped her gain some perspective on her occasional experiences of anger. Now she knows that caregivers should "not be embarrassed or ashamed or feel they don't love the person they're caring for just 'cause they're ready to kill them!" (In chapter 4, we say more about the benefits of social support for caregivers.)

Practical and Economic Demands

Your spouse's physical limitations may make it necessary to modify your home environment. You may need to install a wheelchair ramp, widen doorways, or put grab bars in the shower stall. If your spouse is unable to climb stairs, you may need to make more extensive modifications to your home or even move to a different house or apartment. These modifications may be trying for both of you because of disruptions to your home and your routine and the economic stress of construction or moving. Economic losses are significant for some couples, especially when the stroke survivor is unable to work and the caregiving spouse must take a leave from work or give up employment altogether to provide daily care. Extraordinary medical bills may add to this burden, as health insurance usually covers only part of the high cost of medical care, hospitals, and rehabilitation. (Chapter 6 provides further discussion of insurance benefits and financial planning for health care needs.)

Role Changes

Following a stroke, many couples must change their usual division of labor. Tasks and duties that were previously performed by your spouse, such as driving a car, handling the bills and finances, cooking, shopping, and making social arrangements, may need to be reassigned—to you or someone else. Taking over these responsibilities can be a huge challenge, especially if each of you handled the same tasks over many years of marriage. If you never drove a car or managed the checkbook or planned a meal or a shopping list, learning these tasks for the first time after your spouse's stroke—especially when you are also providing the bulk of his care—is quite a tall order. If you have to take on several new tasks all at once, the challenge is multiplied. If you are an older caregiver, you may find it hard to learn new skills, such as driving, or you may have your own health problems that make it difficult to do these things. If you are a younger, working spouse, you may find it overwhelming to "stretch" your schedule and add more responsibilities to your own already busy week.

When your spouse has a stroke, you are hit with a "double whammy"—adding new caregiving duties to your schedule *and* taking on tasks that your spouse is no longer able to handle. While one side of this coin is increased stress and fatigue for you as a caregiver, the other is feelings of loss or uselessness for your spouse.

Mike and Doris had been married 41 years when Doris had a right-hemisphere stroke resulting in left-side weakness, mild left-neglect, and memory impairment. Since Doris was unable to return to work, Mike retired early and became her full-time caregiver. Before her stroke, Doris and Mike shared almost all the tasks of running a home, but now Mike makes all of their appointments, does all the cooking, and helps Doris with bathing and dressing. They both miss the equal division of chores they had before her stroke. Mike feels the weight of responsibility for her safety and the stress of managing single-handedly the multiple roles they used to share. Doris, in turn, is upset by her inability to contribute. She says, "He does everything. . . . it's like a role reversal. . . . I'm like a bigger child, not a young child, but still there are things I'm not supposed to do. It bothers me that I can't take care of myself."

One of the challenges for many couples after a stroke is to avoid the extremes in which the caregiver "does everything" and feels burdened while the stroke survivor does nothing and feels like a useless lump. Rebalancing roles and responsibilities is necessary so that the spouse who is "holding down the fort" can enjoy a break now and then and the stroke survivor can have the experience of making an adult contribution to the marriage. This can generally be accomplished in one of two ways: by getting more help from outside the marriage (for example, having your family, friends, or a paid employee provide some of your spouse's care or help with cleaning and shopping) or by finding creative ways for the stroke survivor to contribute to the marriage and to the emotional support of the caregiver spouse.

> Wayne had a deep-brain stroke that left him with severe memory loss. Although his physical abilities and speech recovered soon after the stroke, he could not remember things from one day to the next. Initially, his wife, Beth, had to take over everything—driving, bills, cooking, planning appointments—in addition to providing full-time supervision to keep Wayne safe and help him get through his daily activities. But Beth was determined to include Wayne as a partner. Using some of the ideas generated by Wayne's rehab therapists, she taught him how to use calendars, notebooks, and timers to remember his daily chores and appointments. She comments, "Sometimes you get to a point where you say, 'Oh my God, I've got to do *everything* by myself.' But it's not like that. What's better now is instead of it just being me— and him not having *any* memory—now I can at least talk to him and say, 'What do you remember about such and such, what do you think about this?' And I don't have to decide all by myself. He may not remember the conversation the next day, but he's there, in the moment, and he can draw on his past experience. I feel like I can depend on his advice."

For more discussion of strategies for managing role changes and keeping a better balance of the contributions that you and your spouse make to the marriage, see chapters 2 and 5.

Sexuality and Intimacy

Many couples experience changes in their sexual intimacy and satisfaction after stroke. Some changes in sexual function after stroke are biological and are due to the stroke, to other medical conditions (such as diabetes), or to antihypertensive or antidepressant drugs. These medications can cause erectile dysfunction and reduce sexual desire. You may need to make some extra preparations for sexual activity if your spouse has problems with incontinence or uses a urinary catheter, but you can still have an active sex life. In fact, most changes in sexual intimacy after stroke are due to psychological and relationship factors, such as anxiety, fear, depression, lack of communication, or difficulty "switching gears" from caregiver to romantic partner. Fatigue can also affect a person's interest in sex and performance in bed. Many couples find that they need to have sex earlier in the day and to schedule sexual encounters on days when they are rested and not pressed for time.

Like Howie, some spouses fear that sexual intercourse will injure their partner or cause another stroke. Usually, this fear is unfounded. It is unfortunate that many couples are too embarrassed to discuss sex with their physician, because help is available. Some couples simply avoid sexual activity altogether, but avoiding sex is likely to increase frustration and stress in the marriage. Sexual function, sexuality, and methods for improving sexual intimacy after stroke are discussed in detail in chapter 3.

Health Consequences of Caregiving

Caring for your spouse after a stroke can have health consequences for you, the caregiver. The physical, emotional, and economic stresses involved in caregiving cause many caregivers to become socially isolated and depressed and to develop physical health problems. It appears that the negative health effects on caregivers can be caused more by *emotional* stress related to the spouse's repeated hospitalization, suffering, or anticipated decline, than by the physical demands or the amount of time involved in caregiving. One recent study even found that spending a certain amount of time helping your spouse can have a beneficial effect on your health.

Social Isolation

Elaine and Stan had an active social life before his stroke, but they lost many mutual friends because communicating with Stan, who had aphasia, was difficult. Elaine's social contacts with women friends also diminished because, for years after his stroke, she didn't feel comfortable leaving Stan home by himself. She said she feared he would become depressed or that "he'd just sit in front of TV. I couldn't stand the thought of him doing that."

A loss of social activities, hobbies, and recreation is a common consequence of stroke, for both stroke survivors and their spouses, for several reasons. Like Elaine, some caregivers feel guilty about leaving their spouse alone. They may feel they are indispensable for their spouse's well-being or that they must provide their spouse with "quality time" *all* the time. When the stroke survivor needs to have constant care or supervision to make sure he is safe, the spouse's social activities outside the home might be limited because she can't find friends or family who can cover for her. Or she might be worn out by the heavy physical work of caregiving, or emotionally exhausted by caring for a person with depression or severe cognitive impairments and may simply be too tired to go to the movies, play bridge, or have dinner out with friends.

For stroke survivors themselves, depression, apathy, cognitive loss, or feelings of embarrassment about their disability can diminish their desire to engage in the activities they used to enjoy. Like Georgia, some stroke survivors lack the drive to socialize or the initiative necessary to make plans. You may find it easier not to "rock the boat" by pushing your partner to get out and participate in life; but then, like Georgia's husband, Howie, you may find yourself cut off from your friends and the things you like to do. Ways to maintain your own social life and encourage your spouse to be more socially active are discussed in chapters 2, 4, and 5.

Depression

It is not surprising that spouse caregivers are at risk for depression. Unlike Howie's "mild case of the blues," depression is a serious health problem that can cause tremendous personal suffering, make it impossible for the person to function in social situations or at work, and possibly lead to suicide. Feelings of sadness or grief that come and go may be managed by getting support from friends or taking a break from caregiving, but if you are clinically depressed, you probably need treatment with psychotherapy or medication or both.

While we don't know the precise rate of depression for spouse caregivers, it appears that they are at high risk for depression immediately after their spouse's stroke and for as long as one to two years later. Sometimes a life-threatening stroke, like Georgia's, can lead to powerful feelings of anxiety and hopelessness that cause caregiver depression during the very early stages of a spouse's recovery. Later on, depression can result from sadness and grief in the aftermath of a stroke that leaves one's spouse with long-term physical or mental disability. Social isolation, lack of social support, and loss of the pleasure that used to come from enjoyable leisure activities can also contribute to depression for caregivers. Social support seems to protect caregivers from getting depressed. The importance of social support for both you and your spouse is discussed in greater detail in chapters 1 and 4.

Many factors can contribute to depression in spouse caregivers, but the two factors that appear to have the greatest impact are the severity of the stroke and stroke-related emotional or behavioral problems that can alter the relationship between you and your spouse, making caregiving more difficult. (These emotional and behavioral problems are addressed in more detail in chapter 5.) Anything that interferes with communication, especially aphasia, can contribute to depression in both you and your spouse.

Elaine went through a period of depression after Stan's stroke; she felt unable to cope with her feelings of loss, and with Stan's aphasia, it was difficult to have a conversation. As noted earlier, Elaine had high standards for herself as a caregiver and felt guilty if her husband experienced discomfort or boredom. She became isolated and lost her network of supportive friends. Fortunately, Elaine recognized that she was getting depressed and, wisely, asked her doctor for help. After starting to take an antidepressant medication, Elaine felt much better and was able to change her behavior in ways that were beneficial to herself and her husband. (Depression in caregivers and stroke survivors is discussed in chapters 1, 2, and 4.)

Physical Health

Your physical health can easily be affected by strenuous tasks such as helping your spouse transfer in and out of a wheelchair or bed, assisting with bathing, or lifting the wheelchair in and out of the trunk of a car. These actions may be particularly taxing if you are older or already had health problems of your own, and they can increase your risk for injuries and fatigue.

In addition, many caregivers neglect their preventive health care, including checkups, vaccinations, and medical screening tests; they often are fatigued; and they develop new physical symptoms. These physical health risks are closely related to depression and emotional stress. One study, for example, found that emotionally strained older spouse caregivers were more likely to die during the study period than spouses with similar caregiving duties who did not feel emotional strain. Caregivers often don't get enough sleep, eat balanced meals, or get regular exercise. Lack of sleep and poor eating habits contribute to emotional stress and can increase susceptibility to physical illness. Caregivers who break this cycle by finding ways to reduce stress, take care of their own health, and get outside support when it is needed can be good caregivers without sacrificing their own well-being. As mentioned earlier, caring for your spouse can actually improve your health—but only if you can reduce the psychological pain and distress that you experience in dealing with your spouse's illness and recovery. Strategies for enhancing your physical health and well-being are addressed in more detail in chapter 4.

Stroke, Caregiving, and Marriage

Because it often involves changes in thinking, emotion, and behavior, as well as physical disability, a stroke presents a challenge for any marriage. After a stroke, both you and your spouse will need time to adjust to many changes in your life, such as altered communication, difficulty with emotional intimacy, and the limited range of activities you can participate in together. As a couple, you will be working to maintain a well-functioning marriage, one that can meet both the special needs of your stroke survivor spouse and your needs as the "healthy" spouse. You will need to be flexible, willing to experiment, and able to adapt in numerous ways.

Some couples will "bounce back" from stroke better than others. If the two of you have been emotionally close, able to work as a team, and mutually supportive, you will be better able to handle changes brought about by a stroke. If you tend to be mentally flexible and adaptable, it may be easier to reconfigure your relationship in a way that you both find meaningful and satisfying. If you have solid connections to extended family and a community, you will have more access to help when needed.

But coping will be more difficult if, before the stroke, you and your spouse had a rigid assignment of roles and responsibilities, if you were not very close emotionally, or if you had little support from your family or community. Sometimes a stroke can be the "last straw" for a couple whose marriage was already "on the rocks," and in such a case, the stroke can lead to divorce or chronic unhappiness. However, while some couples are "naturally" more adaptable, there are methods for coping with stroke that you can learn and practice as a couple, if you have the motivation to improve your marriage—even if you had some marital problems before the stroke. We address these techniques in the coming chapters.

There are also many ways that you as a caregiving spouse can learn to take care of yourself and improve your own health and well-being after your spouse's stroke. Sometimes caregivers are concerned that paying attention to their own needs is selfish, and they think they should focus all their energy on the spouse who is recovering. But if tension is increasing in your relationship, your efforts to help your spouse are not working, or your own health is suffering, you may need to take a time-out to focus on your own needs. Doing so can be helpful not only for you, but for your marriage as well. Relationships benefit from a positive change in either partner, so taking care of yourself will contribute to your spouse's recovery and to the health of your relationship.

After a few weeks of feeling down in the dumps, Howie had to get out of the house. He arranged with his boss to begin working part time and asked Georgia's daughter Suzy to stay with her two days a week. On Suzy's days as a caregiver, she took Georgia shopping and out to lunch. Howie's return to work boosted his self-esteem, and he enjoyed relating to his co-workers. When he was working, Howie didn't worry so much about Georgia; when he did worry, he could reassure himself that she was in good hands with Suzy.

Howie found that he had more energy for Georgia on the days he was home with her, and he began to notice more of the ways she was making progress. As his mood improved, he became more complimentary and playful with Georgia, using humor and affection, instead of nagging, to encourage her to visit with family and go on outings around town. He invited a few of his friends over to play cards one night; Georgia watched TV in the bedroom but joined them for refreshments after the game. This soon became a weekly ritual that they both enjoyed. As Georgia benefited from the support and stimulation of Suzy's regular visits, and Howie enjoyed regular contact with friends, family, and co-workers, both partners were better able to handle stress and focus more energy on improving the quality of their time together.

In the process of adapting to the changes brought about by a stroke, some spouses discover unexpected benefits for their lives as a couple. Sometimes, for example, role changes are a good thing. They can give a couple more time together, and caregivers who learn challenging new tasks can get a big boost in their confidence and self-esteem.

Jim, a self-described "workaholic," found that "forced retirement" and dependence on his wife after his stroke resulted in a closer relationship. Because of Jim's mild cognitive impairments, his wife, Peggy, had to take over the management of their retirement fund. She found that she had a real knack for investing. By making financial decisions that had a positive impact on their future, Peggy felt that she was contributing to the marriage in a new and important way.

Caregiving may also be an opportunity to give something back in return for the support of a particularly attentive or kind spouse, to "balance the books" in a marriage where you felt you were getting the better end of the deal before the stroke.

Pete had "never lifted a finger" at home. His wife, Daisy, did all the cooking and housework, laid out Pete's clothes each night before going to bed, and packed his lunch in the morning. When Pete hurt his back and was home on medical leave for three weeks, Daisy waited on him hand and foot. Pete took Daisy's help for granted until she had a stroke at age 65; when he had to take over all the household chores, Pete realized how much she had done for him all those years. While terribly distressed by Daisy's stroke, Pete felt gratified by the chance to "make good" on his commitment to her, returning the loving care she had given him throughout their long marriage.

Like other sudden life-changing events, a stroke can prompt you to reassess your identity, reexamine the meaning of your life, and reorder your priorities. Many couples go through this process together after a stroke, as each spouse examines the impact of the stroke on his or her life and on their relationship. Stroke may be seen as a "common enemy" that unites a couple in their efforts to solve problems, find social support, and enhance recovery. It can lead to increased emotional closeness and a heightened sense of shared purpose.

For some couples, a stroke stimulates their efforts to change aspects of their lives that they were unhappy with before. During the sometimes long rehabilitation and recovery, many couples completely suspend their normal routine; while this can be frustrating and unnerving, it can also provide a chance to think about changing their lifestyle and habits. One way for couples to cope with the losses following stroke is by doing more of those activities that are still possible for the stroke survivor and by shifting their focus to aspects of their relationship that remain strong after the stroke. Some couples develop greater appreciation for activities that were low on their prestroke priority list, and some develop new interests or hobbies.

Phil was a magazine editor before a left-brain stroke caused aphasia and weakness of his right side. Return to work was impossible, and he and his wife, Louise, were frustrated by their inability to share the hours of conversation they enjoyed before the stroke. After months of "beating their heads against the wall," Louise began to look for other ways to spend time together. They enrolled in a painting class and found that artwork was an enjoyable way to share their inner experiences, without using words. Louise encouraged Phil to join her in other nonverbal activities—taking walks, going to concerts, and visiting museums. Once they stopped trying so hard to *talk,* they expressed themselves more through touching, smiling, gestures, and physical affection. Louise grew to value her "quiet time" with Phil and continued to seek new ways for them to enjoy life together.

Your spouse's stroke has a significant impact on you and on your marriage. Some strains for caregivers are due to the physical and practical demands of providing care, but many are due to the emotional and social stress of adapting to a partner's stroke. Failing to pay attention to your physical health, developing depression, struggling to cope with role changes, and grieving the disruption of sexual intimacy with your spouse are some of the common problems you may face as a caregiver. If you are able to take care of yourself and to encourage your spouse to contribute more to the marriage, caregiving will probably go more smoothly for you. Stroke may just be the spark that sets off positive changes in your relationship with your spouse, and the new skills you learn as a caregiver might give you a boost in self-confidence.

The chapters that follow will help you improve the quality of care you provide for *your spouse,* take better care of *yourself,* and respond more effectively to the impact of stroke on *your marriage.*

CHAPTER 1

The Secret Ingredient

Stroke and Social Support

One of the most valuable things you do for your spouse after a stroke is provide her with steady and reliable support. Practical assistance is a must, but emotional and social support are equally important. This chapter explains how receiving social support—from you and from other people—provides health benefits and improves your spouse's recovery after a stroke. There are several ways to make sure your spouse has adequate social support:

- Give your own support.
- Organize support from friends and family.
- Help your spouse become involved in community events and recreational activities that include social contact and support.

People are social animals. From our beginnings we have lived in family and tribal social groups. Social ties help make sure that we are nurtured and supported during infancy, old age, and illness and help people work together in groups to meet the needs of each individual. Social support is crucial to our physical health and safety and to our psychological well-being.

The benefits of social support for better health, improved recovery, and lower risk of death from serious illnesses have been confirmed by many research studies. Social support plays a role in mental health, as well; people with less support are more dissatisfied with life and more likely to have symptoms of depression or anxiety. It appears that both the *number* of social connections and the *quality* of these connections influence recovery. Although both casual and close relationships promote better health in general, close relationships that are fraught with conflict or tension can be harmful to health.

Healthy behaviors are also influenced by social support. People with less emotional support and those with conflicts in their close relationships are more likely to smoke, abuse alcohol, and overeat, and they are less likely to make use of preventive health care services. People who have positive support from their families or close friends are more likely to follow recommended medical treatment regimens and to engage in healthy behaviors such as exercising and eating healthy foods.

With all these general health benefits, it comes as no surprise that social support from friends, family, and spouses has a positive influence on recovery from stroke.

Family Social Support after Stroke

Social and emotional support plays a vital role in promoting better stroke outcomes, including

- increased rate and extent of recovery,
- reduced risk for poststroke depression,
- greater cognitive improvement,
- less likelihood of needing nursing home care, and
- improved long-term adjustment and quality of life after stroke.

How do we know this? Because numerous studies done over the past 25 years have shown that social support is one of the strongest and most consistent predictors of poststroke functional ability, that is, the ability to walk, talk, eat, dress, bathe, and perform other functions of daily life.

Although the structure of families has changed in recent years, the family remains the primary social unit for our physical nurturance, emotional support, protection, and care. Of course, individual families vary, and some are more successful than others in carrying out these functions. For most people, the family is the main source of social support after a stroke; the majority of stroke survivors return to their families following discharge from the hospital or the rehabilitation center. So the family's ability to fulfill its supportive function has a major impact on stroke recovery.

> I was a family project!—Wayne, stroke survivor

> Everybody's had to pull together. My older son became a very important factor in how this household operates. He's taken on a lot of responsibilities. I couldn't do it without him. And the little one, he helped after school. He knew all about his dad's medications. It was really a family effort; that's the only way we could work it.—Beth, Wayne's wife and caregiver

Wayne had a high degree of social support available to him, not only from his spouse but also from other family members—and even some extended family. If you are able to mobilize this type of family involvement, your spouse will benefit, and so will *you* (more about that in chapter 4). Remember that *your* support of your spouse can go only so far; getting help from the rest of the family is equally important.

Your family's ability to provide quality social support depends in part on its size and structure and in part on how effectively it functions as a system. Family and marital function is hard to measure objectively. But there are some paper-and-pencil tests and structured interviews that are useful for understanding particular family characteristics, such as communication skills and emotional closeness. Research using some of these tests has shown that better family function is linked to a variety of improvements in stroke recovery.

Family Support Increases the Likelihood of Care at Home

First of all, we do not mean to imply by anything we say here that nursing home care is always a bad idea. As we point out in chapter 5, there are times when nursing home care is the best option, either because the stroke survivor has extreme physical limitations, multiple medical problems, or dementia, or because his spouse or family lacks the physical, emotional, or financial resources to manage complex care at home.

For many stroke survivors, simply *having* a spouse, close relative, or "significant other" makes it possible to live at home instead of in a nursing home. If the person has a larger group of friends and family and a higher degree of family involvement, she may be able to live at home even with severe disability. A spouse caregiver's decision about nursing home care for his or her partner after a stroke is influenced by emotional stress and strain more than by the extent of the stroke survivor's physical care needs. And emotional strain is more common for spouses who have no one to help them in providing care. If a stroke survivor with severe impairments is to thrive at home, her spouse must be emotionally resilient and highly motivated, but often that is not enough. The caregiving spouse will usually need help from other family members as well.

Donna's account illustrates the role of extended family support in making it possible for her father to care for his wife at home after a severe stroke:

> The doctors recommended a nursing home for my mother; they didn't think she'd speak or walk again. But Dad was convinced that Mom would get better at home. So my husband and I moved closer to help them out. Mom was incontinent, in a wheelchair, and she couldn't talk. And we were not prepared at all. We just had to assume we could do it. At first we did everything for her; she was like a baby. It was so hard, watching her struggle with every little thing. But gradually she got better. Now, two years later, she's walking and talking. The other evening she came into the kitchen and I said, "Is Dad going to help you with your shower tonight?" And she said, "I already took it myself!"

While Donna's father was the primary caregiver for his wife, Donna and her husband provided the backup care; this team effort made it possible for Donna's father to provide quality care for his wife at home and was a major factor in her recovery.

Family Support Helps Stroke Survivors Follow Their Doctors' Recommendations

> I wanted a big party for my sixtieth birthday, so my husband arranged it—but he watched what I drank! The neurologist had told us, "Alcohol

is poison for you," so he wouldn't let me take a drop.—Lola, stroke survivor

One of the important supports that caregivers provide is making sure that the stroke survivor sticks to the doctor's treatment plans and recommendations—avoiding alcohol and cigarettes, taking the right medications, going to physical therapy or doing an exercise program, following the prescribed diet, and so forth—all in the service of staying healthy and preventing another stroke. Family communication, problem-solving ability, and emotional involvement help stroke survivors adhere to treatment regimens after stroke. And when stroke survivors "stay with the program," they are less likely to develop medical complications or depression and more likely to improve their functional abilities.

Family Support Helps Prevent Depression

Supportive family relationships play a role in preventing depression for stroke survivors. This is very important, since depression is the most common psychological problem after a stroke, and it frequently leads to bad outcomes, including

- poor recovery in self-care activities (bathing, dressing, grooming, eating),
- less involvement in social activities,
- less ability to follow medical treatment regimens, and
- a higher risk of medical complications and death.

A caregiving spouse and a strong marital relationship can help to prevent depression and promote positive outcomes after stroke.

Marital Support and Stroke Outcomes

Spouse support is a powerful aid to stroke recovery for several reasons, including a spouse's ability to improve the stroke survivor's mood and to increase physical and social activity levels. Animal studies reveal that social support can also change what happens in the brain after stroke. In one study, a group of male mice had had experimentally induced strokes. Some of them were placed in cages with females, and others were placed in cages alone. The mice that were placed with the females had less brain swelling after stroke. So in addition to having psychological, physical, and social benefits, your support may also influence your spouse's stroke recovery on the neurological level.

We know that providing effective support for a person after a stroke is important to recovery, but it is difficult to determine ahead of time exactly what support will be effective. And the diversity of individuals and couples means that behaviors or interactions that are experienced as supportive by one person at one time are seen as annoyances by another person or at another time. Providing the "best" kind of support is not always intuitive—or easy—even when you have a good relationship with your spouse. We discuss several issues related to spouse support after a stroke to give you some ideas about how to tweak your relationship and make your interactions with your spouse more beneficial.

Reducing Your Spouse's Risk for Depression

Depression, a common and potentially serious problem that often gets in the way of recovery from stroke, is more common in stroke survivors who have a bad relationship with the person closest to them. When depressed stroke survivors feel that their spouse is not supportive, they have more severe and longer-lasting depressions. This is an area where your knowledge and awareness can make a big difference for your spouse. Becoming familiar with the symptoms of clinical depression is the first step. These symptoms typically include insomnia; loss of appetite; irritability; loss of interest in the person's usual activities; inability to experience pleasure; pervasive feelings of sadness, worthlessness, or hopelessness; and thoughts of death or suicide. Knowing that poststroke depression can be a serious problem for your spouse (and for yourself; see chapter 4), you may be able to take steps to prevent it. Closely monitoring your spouse's mood and getting him involved in enjoyable activities are two ways you can "nip depression in the bud."

I work very hard to keep Stan from getting depressed. He was extraordinarily busy, with his own business, computers. He was a painter, liked rock climbing . . . so I try to keep him busy now. I've heard horror stories about what happens to stroke survivors who get depressed. And besides, if he gets depressed, then I'll get depressed!—Elaine, wife and caregiver

"Tuning in" to the activities, social contacts, and communications that improve your spouse's self-image and confidence is helpful. With your encouragement, your spouse may be able to take up social and other activities where she left off before her stroke. You may need to be creative about finding new things for your spouse to do and discovering new ways to communicate your positive feelings for him. Modeling an optimistic outlook for your spouse and letting him know that you have hope for his recovery may also play a role in enhancing his mood and preventing depression.

The first few weeks after rehab, he did feel depressed and very frustrated. He would just say "Whatever you want," maybe in part because he couldn't express himself. He was very passive. I couldn't understand why, but I just assumed that mentally he would get better. I tried to make life as normal as possible for all of us.—Toni, Luis's wife and caregiver

One way to keep things "normal" is to create expectations that your spouse will do as much as she can. While the expectations need to be realistic (reasonable, given your spouse's abilities), it is helpful to give your spouse a gentle nudge to try doing some of the things she enjoyed and was good at before her stroke. Like Luis, many stroke survivors become passive after a stroke or are afraid to test their abilities.

Toni found a way to push Luis, he says, "past my comfort zone. It was good for me to be pushed! She expected me to do most of what I did before. She had parties at our house and got me dancing again, doing things for fun. When we went camping for the first time after my stroke, she went to the camp store with my daughter and told me to set up the tent! And I did, with one hand."

But not all spouses are able to use Toni's approach of "pushing" their partner to socialize, go on trips, and be more physically independent. You may be afraid to encourage your spouse's independence because of concerns for his physical safety. Or you might not have the support to cope with your spouse's depression, might be unsure of how to help, or might lack the mental energy necessary to pull him out of a funk.

> Doris has had bouts of depression since her stroke. She is embarrassed by her disability and often avoids socializing. Mike finds it difficult to get Doris involved in activities outside the house or to find things for her to do at home that would boost her confidence. Because he is nervous about her safety and fearful that she might fall, he tends to watch her closely and often jumps in to do things for her rather than let her attempt difficult tasks. Although Doris appreciates Mike's devotion and care, she continues to struggle with feelings of uselessness related to her "inability to do much of anything."

You may find, like Mike, that an overwhelming sense of responsibility for your partner's safety prevents you from encouraging her to do the things that would improve her mood, such as using her physical and social skills. If so, you might benefit from attending a caregiver support group or getting professional counseling to lessen your anxiety and make you more comfortable with letting your spouse engage in meaningful activities. Sometimes in caregiving, as in parenting, "less is more," and it is helpful to know when to "let go" of your partner and allow her to take reasonable risks to experience life to the fullest.

Instrumental versus Emotional Support

This brings us to a discussion of two important types of social support. The first is *instrumental*, or practical; it includes

- helping your spouse physically (such as with bathing, eating, or walking),
- doing necessary chores for him (such as cooking, shopping, driving, and paying bills), or
- making changes in the physical environment to enhance her function (such as installing grab bars in the shower, installing a ramp, or creating a calendar or notebook to help her remember things).

The second type is *emotional* support, activities such as

- talking and listening;
- expressing concern, affection, and encouragement;

- trying to motivate or help your spouse to solve problems; and
- spending time with your spouse doing enjoyable things like playing a game, eating dinner at a restaurant, or visiting friends.

Instrumental support is absolutely necessary when your spouse has physical or cognitive impairments that limit his ability to function independently. It includes everything that you, or others, do to help him meet his basic needs—providing physical care, keeping him safe, and maintaining his health. While instrumental support is necessary for *any* recovery, emotional support is the "secret ingredient" necessary for the *best possible* recovery.

High levels of emotional support lead to better recovery after a stroke, and support is most effective when it is seen by the stroke survivor as meeting her particular emotional needs. In particular, *empathy,* your ability to see things from the other person's perspective, or to understand how he is feeling, is especially helpful in promoting stroke recovery.

> Stan was unable to drive for six years after his stroke. Elaine recognized how confined he felt and encouraged him to take a driver training class for stroke survivors, which he completed successfully. "He was so happy with his new independence," she says. When Elaine thought Stan was losing his sense of direction, she bought him a GPS and taught him how to use it. Her empathy for the feelings of freedom and pleasure that Stan had earlier experienced through driving provided the motivation for her to help him regain his driving skills.

One of the most difficult issues you face as a spouse caregiver is balancing instrumental support for your spouse on the one hand and emotional support on the other. You may experience some conflict between the need to protect and care for your spouse and the need to encourage your spouse to become more independent and competent.

When it comes to instrumental support, there can be too much of a good thing; excessive instrumental support can stand in the way of your spouse's attempts to "spread his wings" and limit his potential independence. Although therapists often determine during rehabilitation that stroke survivors are *capable* of doing things such as cooking, washing dishes, or walking, they don't actually *do* these things once they get home. Similarly, some stroke survivors who are physically and mentally able to go out to social activities in the community choose instead to stay home. While depression, cognitive deficits, and decreased self-awareness can prompt a stroke survivor to do less than she is able to, the interaction between you and your spouse also plays a part in whether she actually *uses* her capabilities at home, once her rehabilitation program is completed.

If your spouse has significant mobility or cognitive problems, you may initially have to provide intensive instrumental *and* emotional support. But it is easy to get in the habit of helping your spouse with numerous everyday tasks, and you can lose track of his slow progress and improvements. If you continue to assist him in the same way you did before he made these improvements, you can provide *too much* help, making him overly dependent. Try to stay aware of your spouse's progress, perhaps by keeping a journal or giving him frequent chances to try things on his own. This will help you see when it is time to stop providing so much help and instead to start coaxing him to do more for himself.

Your spouse's recovery will progress more smoothly if you can modify the intensity and type of support you provide, depending on changes in his particular limitations and abilities.

Beth found that she needed to adjust her support strategy as her husband Wayne's recovery progressed. Initially, she was very focused on his safety and found that she became, as she put it, "bossy, because I had to be. That's what he needed at the time. I was so afraid he would fall down the basement steps [because he couldn't remember his limitations]." As Wayne's self-awareness and balance improved, Beth began to focus more on ways to structure his day so he could stay active and use as many of his skills as possible. "The biggest challenge is filling his time, keeping him engaged, but we've done well with it." Every day their family calendar is filled with activities, and although he continues to have memory problems, Wayne enjoys participating in a variety of social events and household chores.

Problems arise when a caregiver becomes overprotective. This often happens when he becomes so completely involved in his helping role that he fears he will no longer be valued or needed when his spouse recovers. Paradoxically, caregivers who are exceptionally caring, competent, and high-functioning people seem to be prone to developing an overprotective attitude. If you are doing your job extremely well, it can be very hard to compromise. When you know you can make a superb meal for your spouse, or pick out a color-coordinated outfit for her, it is hard to stand by and let her do the same things far from perfectly. But when you insist on things being "just so" or are afraid to let your spouse take any risks, you can unintentionally stand in the way of her functional recovery, discouraging her from solving problems herself.

> Doris notes that although she is able to do some cooking, "It's hard with one hand. Sometimes it's easier for my husband to just do it." Doris says her husband also helps her get dressed—although she is able to do it herself—"because I tend to put things on inside out. It doesn't bother me, but it bothers him."

It is difficult to watch your spouse experience frustration when trying new things, and it can be frustrating for you when the results of his efforts are not immediately obvious. Watching your spouse struggle with things that used to be easy can make you feel highly anxious or uncomfortable. Sometimes getting a break from caregiving, talking to understanding friends, or attending a caregiver group can help you override these feelings, and you can begin to give your spouse *more* emotional support by providing *less* practical assistance. Staying involved in outside social activities (such as work, hobbies, volunteering, and other valuable roles you play within your family) may help you tolerate frustration, avoid becoming overly wrapped up in the caregiver role, and reduce your tendency to overprotect your spouse.

> As Stan has developed an independent social life, Elaine has had to relinquish the sense of control she developed during years of being "in charge of everything." She says she feels "more frustration, now that he's going out on his own. I'll say to him 'tell me about your day.' I want to promote conversation, but he can't tell me—or I don't get it [because of his aphasia]. It's a new problem because before I was with him 24 hours a day. Now it's all guesswork. I can't share it with him." Even though she sometimes feels excluded or uneasy about Stan's

ability to manage his new experiences, Elaine continues to encourage his independence.

In some cases the stroke survivor's personality or the speed of her recovery leaves no room for overprotective caregiving. It may be your spouse who takes the lead in pushing both of you along in adapting to her stroke and to her progress in recovery.

Lucy recalls that her husband was "very controlling. When I came home after my rehab, he wanted to do everything, like I couldn't even move without him! When I started going out by myself, he wanted me to call home every half hour. But I'm very obstinate and persistent; I like my freedom. After a while he saw I would be OK, and he adjusted."

In other cases, the caregiver's experience of fatigue or boredom with a particular caregiving task can be a clue that it's time to either take a break or try a different approach.

Janet helped Eli with his speech therapy practice for many months with good results, but then it started to "get old." She says, "I had experience as a teacher in the past, and I was like his teacher/study partner. It was actually very enjoyable at times. But sometimes I'd get tired of all this helping."

If you are feeling the strain of helping with a specific activity, consider stepping back from it to see if your spouse has reached a plateau in his progress and needs a break or, alternatively, if he is able to move ahead on his own without your help.

Getting Your Spouse to Participate in Social Activities

Participating in a variety of social, leisure, and recreational activities is one of the hallmarks of recovery after stroke. Regardless of your spouse's level of physical, cognitive, or functional recovery, her involvement in these activities—to whatever degree is possible—will enable her to reap the benefits of social support from the broader community, which are so important for her psychological and social recovery.

Rita takes her husband Paul to the movies and out to lunch. "It's all within walking distance," she says, "so I can wheel him there myself."

Even though he doesn't eat (because he has dysphagia and uses tube feedings), "he still likes to go with me and be around other people." She finds that Paul often engages in lively conversations with people they meet in the neighborhood, and the positive responses he gets from them are a great boost to his morale.

Getting involved in social activities provides much more than social and emotional support. It also offers opportunities to stimulate mental functions (such as memory, language, and problem-solving), learn and practice new skills, maintain and build physical stamina, and . enjoy both familiar and new experiences. Participating in social activities reduces feelings of sadness and isolation and enhances recovery across the board.

Unfortunately, many stroke survivors withdraw from social activities, even when they are physically capable of participating. They may feel embarrassed by their need for assistance or because they have trouble communicating. Or they may be sad, depressed, anxious, or lacking in initiative.

One of the most helpful things you can do is encourage your spouse to get back into the kinds of activities he enjoyed before his stroke—or explore new ones that may be more compatible with his new abilities and limitations. If he is embarrassed or afraid of taking on new social challenges, look for group activities at first. Stroke clubs often include group social hours, holiday parties, and day trips. Athletic associations for people with disabilities have swimming, golf, and other types of sports and recreation on the calendar (see the Resources section at the end of this book for more ideas). Once your spouse is comfortable in such circles, she may be able to venture into activities outside the stroke survivors' community.

Having a social life, both individually and as a couple, is likely to enhance your quality of life. If you can help your spouse to get back into his own social and leisure activities outside the home after stroke, it will benefit both of you.

Elaine found that once Stan was able to have an independent social life, she was able to take time for herself, too, returning to art classes and lunches with friends. At the same time, she and Stan continued to go out together and to keep up their friendships with other couples.

Beth experienced a sense of relief when Wayne became involved in the men's club at church and started going out for breakfast and meeting friends on his own. She was able to pick up her "girls' night out" and even take occasional overnight trips. As a couple, she and Wayne gradually returned to the full social life they had enjoyed prior to the stroke. She reports, "He does all kinds of things—we're both involved at church, we go bowling, roller skating, we see friends, go to dinner and movies, shows. We play golf together. And Wayne can travel alone, too. He's even taken plane trips with our nine-year-old son. He goes along on school field trips. And he goes to the stroke support group every month."

Social support is essential for people recovering from stroke. Family, friends, and community are all important sources of support. As a spouse, you provide the most reliable and intense support, and you are at the center of the support network. Your spouse may need your help to access the many social supports that are available. In your relationship with your spouse, be aware of keeping a balance between practical and emotional support, and avoid overprotecting her. Subsequent chapters explore how you can increase your spouse's independence and ability to contribute to your marriage. And we will look at how you can make the best use of social supports from your extended family, friends, and community to take better care of yourself as well as your spouse.

Practical Tips for Supporting Your Spouse

- You should not be the *only* source of social support for your spouse. Try to involve other family and friends in supporting him, and encourage his involvement in community social events.

- If your spouse has complex care needs, you may need to get help from others to care for her at home.

- Be aware of signs of depression in your spouse.

- Set up expectations for your spouse: let him know that you expect him to do what he is *able* to do.

- Avoid overprotecting your spouse by providing too much practical help.

- Emotional support is essential. Be sure to listen to your spouse and try to understand her experiences and needs. Talk to her and express your feelings. Spend time doing enjoyable things with her.

- Stay involved in social activities with your spouse.

CHAPTER 2

You Are the One

*Balancing the Roles of Caregiver
and Marriage Partner*

Wayne and Beth had a fulfilling marriage and family life; they had two sons. Beth managed a trucking company, while Wayne worked as an attorney. They were an active family, involved in church, sports, cultural events, traveling, and volunteer work. Although he had never been seriously ill, Wayne had high cholesterol and high blood pressure, smoked, and worked long hours.

After his stroke, Wayne was in the ICU and received acute care for a month, followed by a month of inpatient rehabilitation. On the day he returned home, he had a second, milder stroke. Initially, he was "very, very weak, could barely move one side." The strokes had damaged areas in both sides of his brain, resulting in weakness of all four limbs, severe memory impairment, and poor awareness of his disabilities. When he came home, Beth experienced, she says, "the fear factor. I was so afraid that he'd get sick again. And he was under my care. I was terrified—afraid of the future and the enormity of the task. How do you help someone get their life back? It's a daunting responsibility."

Although Wayne's physical strength and mobility improved rapidly, his memory and cognitive deficits initially made it unsafe for him to move around without supervision. Wayne recalls that in the first year, his family "had to tell me how to do everything. They had to tell me when I could go to the bathroom!" Before his stroke, Wayne had paid bills, worked on home projects, and made financial decisions for the family. After his stroke, Beth had to take over these tasks, make all decisions related to running the home, ensure that Wayne took the right medications, and take him to doctor's appointments and therapies. She also became the primary breadwinner and took on a much greater portion of the child-rearing responsibilities. "It was hard for me to recognize all the things he couldn't do, and figure out how to get around it. I was fearful of dropping one of the balls—the kids, him, work, the house." Beth began to feel overwhelmed.

Like so many other spouse caregivers, Beth struggled with complicated feelings about her dual roles as a wife and intimate partner on the one hand and a caregiver and "manager" on the other. Before Wayne's stroke, Beth and Wayne had shared the responsibilities of working, parenting, and running the household. They had created a true partnership, which included emotional intimacy, shared values and interests, commitment to their family and community, and a feeling that they could each depend on the other. This was seriously disrupted by Wayne's stroke, which left him dependent on Beth for many of his basic needs and placed Beth fully "in charge" of Wayne's life.

Beth felt personally responsible for Wayne's safety and his recovery, yet she was uneasy about suddenly having to make all the major decisions for both of them; and she feared that her "bossiness" made her less desirable as a wife and lover. While Beth began to feel stuck in her role as "bossy caregiver," Wayne was in danger of slipping into the passive role of "patient/care recipient" and getting depressed or apathetic. Beth began to lose her independent sense of self as she became absorbed in the caregiver role.

Getting Stuck in the Caregiver Role

Even though your situation is different from Wayne and Beth's, you may feel similarly bogged down. Because taking care of your spouse creates some unavoidable inequalities in your relationship, constant juggling is required to keep the balance between your role as a caregiver and the reciprocal partnership role you play in your marriage. There are pitfalls in the care-providing process that can lead to feelings of being trapped in an all-encompassing caregiver role.

Fear is one emotion that can cause you to allow caregiving to claim an unfair share of your attention. You may feel so frightened by the idea of "something happening" to your spouse—a fall, another stroke, an emotional upset—that you are reluctant to let her try to do things that she did before the stroke or to try new things to see what she is capable of doing. Despite the difficulty of taking on total responsibility for someone else, that might still seem easier than dealing with the potential danger of letting your spouse try new things on his own—even though his success would take some of the burden off your shoulders. If you worry too much about your spouse, you can fall into the habit of continually protecting him and doing things for him, even things he could do for himself. Rather than "helping" and "protecting" him, you may be making him more dependent and less able to assume new responsibilities. You may find yourself continuing to do it all for much longer than you really need to—and feeling that you have painted yourself into a corner.

Another potential problem is guilt; you may think you are not living up to your commitment or not being a good caregiver if you "push" your spouse to do anything for herself. Many people feel guilty because their spouse had a stroke and they did not; this feeling, though understandable, is utterly unwarranted. Still, feelings of guilt may make you feel that your spouse's needs are *always* more important than your own. Guilt is a very uncomfortable feeling; if you feel guilty much of the time (or if your spouse is actively "laying on the guilt" by reminding you of his disadvantages), you are more likely to put all of your energy into caregiving, to try to ease your guilt. If you feel that your spouse got a "raw deal" because of his stroke, it may seem as if your extra caregiving efforts will somehow equalize things between you. But if you constantly ignore your own needs in favor of your spouse's, you will gradually come to resent him, which simply reverses the emotional imbalance—*you* begin to see *yourself* as the one who is "owed," because you are trying to carry an impossible burden. This is a bad situation that can cause you to make poor decisions for your spouse or to pull back from your spouse and your caregiving responsibilities in a way that is harmful to him.

Some spouses find that there are advantages to the caregiver role; this feeling can contribute to getting "stuck" in that role for an extended period. Caring for your spouse might give you a terrific sense of pride and accomplishment. Taking over responsibilities that were once your spouse's duties gives you the opportunity to learn new skills, and it can give you a wonderful feeling of competence. You may feel more self-confident and enjoy having more control over planning and decision making in your marriage and family. It may be difficult to surrender that newfound control, especially if, before your spouse's stroke, you felt unsure of your abilities or your spouse was the major decision maker. You may fear that if you allow her to regain a more equal role in the marriage, you will lose ground in these areas of personal growth. The challenge is to find ways *other than caregiving* to increase your skills and self-esteem; then you can continue to experience these positive changes in yourself without feeling a need to limit your spouse's contributions to the relationship.

Some caregivers get stuck in the role of "super-caregiver" because they feel the need to justify their decisions surrounding caregiving. This may be the case, for example, if you quit your job or gave up other valuable activities or relationships to provide full-time care for your spouse. It may become important to leave no room for doubt (in your own mind or others' minds) that your spouse needs you and that you did the "right" thing. Or if you were a homemaker who was financially dependent on your spouse, you might feel an obligation to take exemplary care of him now that he is unable to work. Either of these situations can tempt a person to become overly invested in the caregiving role and neglect her own needs and other aspects of her relationship with her spouse.

For some people caregiving can become a crutch, an excuse for not tackling other responsibilities that are less appealing. Rita, for example, recalled that her husband's care needs gave her a good "reason" for not exercising—something she dreaded but needed to do for her own health. Because caregiving is generally seen by others as a noble endeavor, it can be easy to use your caregiving duties as a way to avoid unwanted obligations, or to put off dealing with difficult personal problems or making decisions.

Caregiving pitfalls can occur even in the best of marriages. Having mixed or changing feelings about the place of caregiving in your relationship is to be expected, so it makes sense to reassess your situation from time to time to see how you (and your spouse) are managing the caregiving–care receiving exchanges in your marriage, and all the rest of the marriage, too—partnership, friendship, and intimacy. It may be helpful to ask yourself the following questions:

- Can I safely and comfortably give up some parts of my caregiver role?
- Do I need to pay more attention to other roles I play in my marriage?
- Can my spouse contribute more to achieving a better balance in our relationship?

If you have become mired in caregiving and the rest of your marriage is taking a backseat, you may need to ask yourself how you can get "unstuck."

Getting Unstuck

How can you balance the dual roles of caregiver and marriage partner? First, *create opportunities for your spouse to contribute* her fair share to the marriage. Second, *get help with caregiving* from outside the marriage—don't try to do all the caregiving yourself. Third, because caregiving can so easily consume your energies, direct more attention to *enjoying a shared social life and doing other enjoyable activities together.*

Create Opportunities for Your Spouse to Contribute

Good marital relationships are based on give and take and on interdependence. Spouses in good marriages negotiate how they will achieve these conditions in their relationship. When your spouse has a stroke and you become his caregiver, the balance of give and take will necessarily shift, at least temporarily. Depending on the extent of your spouse's impairments, the shift will result in more or less imbalance, with you giving more and your spouse receiving more in numerous areas. Restoring 50-50 reciprocity in your relationship may not be possible; in fact, like most couples, you and your spouse probably contributed unequal amounts of give and take in certain areas *before* the stroke. A more important goal in making a marriage work is for each spouse to contribute an equal or greater amount in *some* important areas (or at some point in time) to "balance the books" because he or she receives more in another area (or at another time).

When caregiving becomes the main event in your relationship, your marriage can become increasingly unbalanced over time. Your previous agreements may not hold because your spouse is now unable to do things that you both agreed she would do, long before the stroke. To get unstuck from the inherently unequal positions of caregiver and care receiver, the two of you need to periodically negotiate *new* agreements. Your new agreements will take into consideration both her new impairments *and* her capacities for giving. She must be allowed to contribute more to the relationship and to meeting *your* needs, and you must be allowed to relinquish some of your caregiving duties if they put an unfair burden on you. Depending on your spouse's level of physical and mental ability, your agreements may include opportunities for you to receive more support or enjoyment from activities outside of the marriage. "Having a life" beyond caregiving will help you continue to be a good caregiver without feeling resentful and deprived.

Even if your spouse has significant cognitive impairments, you can probably find ways for him to contribute more, and you can negotiate new agreements that result in a better balance of caregiving and other marital roles. As Beth and Wayne's story (which continues below) illustrates, when your spouse cannot participate fully in the process of negotiation because of cognitive impairments, you may have to take the lead in drafting new agreements that are better for you, your spouse, and your relationship. In essence, you may have to create the conditions that allow your spouse to contribute to the practical and emotional aspects of your marriage. This will involve an initial investment of energy as you devise strategies to increase your spouse's independence and work to improve his communication, reasoning, memory, and expression of emotions. The effort will be worthwhile, though, if he can start contributing more to the marriage and you can enjoy a better balance between being a caregiver and being a partner.*

---

*In rare cases, your spouse may be too impaired to make agreements, or even to understand what the relevant issues are in your relationship. This situation, discussed in detail in chapter 5, is one in which caregiving can become a "one-way street" if your spouse is unable to give more in *any* area of your relationship. You may choose to continue as a caregiver—but perhaps do less of the caregiving yourself—while seeking support and companionship through relationships with other people.

The agreements we are describing are typically oral and informal rather than formal written documents. But they carry weight and are important to the success of your marriage. Some caregivers, with more or less input from their spouses, are able to renegotiate these agreements on their own and make successful changes through a process of trial and error. But many caregivers get guidance from a professional counselor or psychologist who helps them generate ideas to move the process along and make it less stressful for everyone. A psychologist who is familiar with stroke and its consequences can address the specific cognitive, emotional, or other problems your spouse is experiencing and can recommend treatments or changes in routines that will maximize her ability to contribute to the marriage.

Counseling was extremely helpful for Beth as she created ways to bring Wayne back to his role as a marriage partner.

Beth recalls that when they took their first family vacation after Wayne's stroke, "I was falling apart. I remember thinking, 'This whole family's on edge. We have got to get some help!' I knew then that if I didn't do something, it was not going to be good!" Beth located a clinical social worker through her local Stroke Association chapter. "She was instrumental in showing me that Wayne was getting better and I could let him try to do things, see where he was improving. She became our go-to person. She pointed me in so many helpful directions." The social worker put Beth and Wayne in touch with a cognitive rehabilitation therapist, to help them find ways for Wayne to function better in spite of his memory deficits.

Working with the therapist, Beth created a large wall calendar listing all of Wayne's and the family's daily activities and appointments. Wayne carries a day-planner book, where he writes all his own appointments and a daily to-do list. He wears a watch with an alarm that beeps hourly, a reminder for him to check his planner. When Wayne started driving again, two years after his stroke, Beth helped him make directions cards for all the places he drives to on a regular basis. He keeps these in a small spiral-bound notebook and refers to them before every trip. Beth helps Wayne figure out how to handle new information so he can do more things for himself and for her; for example, she writes down the code for his ATM card in several places and makes shopping lists.

These strategies take some planning and effort "on the front end," but they have made it possible for Wayne to do the family's grocery shopping, get money from the bank, drive to his own therapy appointments, make his own lunch or go out to eat while Beth is at work, carpool the kids, and keep an active social calendar. They created a structured system that allows Wayne to gradually take on more responsibilities as he improves, and although they both need to spend time maintaining the system, Beth feels that the practical and emotional benefits for her and the marriage far outweigh the time spent to make it possible.

"He's improved so much," she says. "It's bolstered my confidence. I feel like I can depend on him." Wayne has gradually been able to take on more parenting responsibilities. "He's very engaged and involved now with the kids, with the family. We're constantly talking about the kids, what they're doing. And he's my partner. It wasn't really a family when he wasn't really *in* it—but he's coming back."

Beth's new confidence in Wayne's ability to effectively and consistently use the strategies they've developed means that she can rely on him in important ways; she no longer feels that she's doing it all by herself. Wayne is increasingly able to provide emotional support for Beth, and they enjoy their free time together, socializing with others or hanging out at home. Wayne is aware that it is Beth's efforts, in large part, that make it possible for him to be an active partner in their relationship, and he is committed to helping Beth and making a significant contribution to their marriage and family. He notes: "Stroke throws everything for a loop. And if you're not paying attention, it'll all fall apart. You try to grow closer, try to become stronger. You have to be involved as much as possible. And just be as helpful as you can." Although Beth continues to be a caregiver for Wayne, they no longer function as *only* caregiver and care recipient—they feel like friends and partners again.

Like Beth, Toni helped keep the balance in her relationship with Luis by creating opportunities for him to take part in household projects and decisions. Although Luis had been a take-charge person before, after his stroke he had a tendency to sit back and let Toni run the show. But Toni sensed that Luis was still capable of making an intellectual contribution, even though he had some difficulty communicating. She made a point of consulting him on all major decisions, making sure to get his opinions and to tap into his knowledge and expertise, drawing him back into partnership in their marriage. She also found that little things could go a long way toward increasing Luis's independence and contributions. For example, she encouraged him to use the special gadgets his occupational therapists gave him—a button-hook, a rocker knife, and one-handed scissors. While these aids often end up stuck in a drawer or closet, never to be seen again, they can help stroke survivors become more independent in dressing, eating, and hobby activities. Pointing out how these tools could make it easier for Luis to do things for himself was part of renegotiating an agreement with Luis. As his strength and language ability improved, Luis became increasingly involved in all aspects of their marriage and family life; eventually, he was able to resume volunteering and then part-time work.

Changing roles can be difficult for couples, even those who are not dealing with the aftermath of stroke. If a wife wants her husband to share more of the cooking duties, she may find it difficult to encourage his attempts if the results are not "up to her standards." Similarly, a husband who complains that his wife never pays the bills may be flustered if she takes on the job but files receipts according to a different system from his—or without any system at all. Many spouses abandon their attempts to change roles, whether disability is an issue or not.

When your spouse has a stroke, her attempts to take over tasks may get the job done, but not in the way you want it done. As you are creating and reinforcing opportunities for your spouse to help, you may need to revise your expectations, or even lower your standards temporarily, so you can appreciate whatever help she can offer—even if it takes her longer or she does it less carefully than you would like. As Vera's story illustrates, any task your spouse can take on is one less task *you* have to do.

Vera's husband Joey had a stroke in his mid-thirties. At that time, she says, "We both lost our independence. Joey had to go on disability and I had to take a leave from my job. He went from being the primary breadwinner and this totally energetic, outgoing guy to sitting in a wheelchair and needing help with everything. He couldn't work or do for himself, and I couldn't work or do anything else I used to—like run to the gym on Saturday morning or go out for a drink with my friends after work. We *both* felt trapped. But Joey's very motivated and he hated sitting around. So as soon as he was able, I would set him up in the morning and he would do all his own shaving and dressing. It took him forever and I really had to fight the urge to step in. But then it dawned on me that if I let him alone and he took an hour to get ready, well, that was an hour that I could be doing something else. We started experimenting with other things, like having him fold the laundry, load the dishwasher, and set the table. I had to give myself an 'attitude adjustment' because sometimes the laundry was a little sloppy or the silverware was all on one side of the plate—but then I realized, who cares!—at least I don't have to do it myself. When I felt tempted to say something critical, I'd just bite my tongue and say 'Thanks, honey!' Joey got more confident and wanted to help more, and I really felt like we were sharing our lives again."

By experimenting with a variety of tasks to see what he was capable of doing, Vera and Joey were able to negotiate new agreements about Joey's share of the household responsibilities, taking into account his ongoing limitations as well as his abilities. Vera recognized that by being a hovering "nervous Nellie," she would not only prevent Joey from doing what he could do for himself and her, but also deprive herself of time she could spend on her own needs. This combination—finding ways for Joey to contribute while being more concerned with having time to "do her own thing" and less concerned about making sure that Joey's accomplishments were perfect—allowed Vera and Joey to begin sharing more than just caregiving exchanges.

Get Help with Caregiving from Outside Your Marriage

Another way to redirect more of your time and energy toward other aspects of your marriage is to accept assistance from others for some of your caregiving responsibilities. Many spouse caregivers find that spending hours each day providing assistance with activities such as dressing, bathing, cooking, and driving not only takes time away from other activities they would like to enjoy with their wife or husband; it also leads to physical exhaustion that wrecks the "mood" for sharing intimate conversations, physical affection, or even a quiet dinner with their spouse. If some of these care tasks can be handled by a part-time aide or another family member, you will have more time and energy to pursue more emotionally rewarding activities with your spouse.

> When Luis returned home from rehab, his mother flew in from out of state to help. She provided the daily supervision that he initially required, helped him get dressed, prepared breakfast and lunch, and encouraged him to practice his daily physical and speech therapy exercises. Because Luis was cared for at home, Toni could return to work full time, without worrying about his safety. "I was still a caregiver," she says; "there were even times when I was at work, and his mom would call and say, 'He wants *you*,' and I'd have to come home." But most days, Toni enjoyed her work without interruption or worry. When she came home at night, she was happy to see Luis and had the energy to relate to him as a wife, lover, and companion. Because his mother was available to help Luis in the early morning, Toni was also able to continue her daily routine of running for exercise. Running was "a huge destressor," and it helped Toni keep in shape and continue feeling that she was a physically attractive partner for Luis.

Toni could balance her roles as caregiver, wife, mother, and businesswoman largely because she had help with caregiving from outside the marriage. You may not be able to have a relative helping full time, as Toni did, but it may be possible to have some respite care, relying on a relative part time or hiring a caregiver for a few hours a week. Any relief you can get from the day in, day out tasks of caregiving can help you focus more on your marriage as a source of companionship and intimacy and maintain other activities that are essential to your sense of identity and self-esteem. In Toni's case, having her mother-in-law's help also meant that she could return to her job and support the family financially while Luis was unable to work. If you are employed outside the home, it may be economically essential for you to continue working, and getting help from another family member or hired caregiver may be a necessity. But even if the additional income is not essential, or if you work only a few hours a week, your work life may provide a valuable counterbalance to your role as a caregiver. Work can increase your feelings of effectiveness and self-confidence and contribute importantly to your enjoyment of life and sense of identity as an individual.

> When Vera needed to return to work, the social worker at Joey's rehabilitation center helped her locate a professional caregiver who could work a few days a week and whose rates were reasonable. The hired caregiver drove Joey to his therapies; took him out for walks, shopping, and other errands; and helped Vera by starting dinner and doing light cleaning. Both Vera and Joey felt liberated by this arrangement—Vera could get out of the house and work, and Joey, with the help of the paid caregiver, could take on the responsibilities of shopping, picking up clothes from the cleaners, and going to the bank. With fewer chores to do in the evenings, Vera and Joey could enjoy having dinner and relaxing together, and on the weekends they spent time with friends, went to the movies, and, Vera said, just "started to go about our lives together, doing the things we always liked, as much as we could."

Share Enjoyable Hobbies, Social Activities, and Romance

When you and your spouse devote time to enjoying social and recreational activities and activities that encourage intimacy and romance, you move toward a better balance in your relationship. Sharing hobbies and leisure activities at home and a social life in the community helps couples to be friends and companions. Social, leisure, recreational, and romantic pursuits are like glue, holding you and your spouse together emotionally. If you keep these parts of your marriage alive, your relationship is less likely to become one-sided and dominated by caregiving.

> From the moment Luis came home from the rehabilitation hospital, Toni concentrated her efforts on having fun with him. She hosted parties at home where music and dancing were part of the evening's entertainment, and she took Luis out to see friends. These shared social events and activities helped to take the focus off Luis as a "patient" and Toni as a "caregiver" and allowed them to quickly regain the sense of romance and fun that was central to their lives together.

Every couple's interests are different. As much as you can, continue the types of leisure activities that you and your spouse enjoyed before the stroke—such as dancing, golfing, playing cards, or taking day trips. Depending on the physical and cognitive consequences of your spouse's stroke, you may need to find new or alternative activities that match his current capabilities. Computer technology has created many leisure opportunities for people with and without disabilities. Participating in chat rooms and social networking sites, corresponding by e-mail or videophone with far-away family members, buying and selling items online, and playing computer games are all outlets for someone who is unable to engage in more physical activities or to leave home. Computer games have the added benefit of stimulating a person's attention, memory, and cognitive function.

Once formal physical therapy is completed, going to exercise classes, a swimming pool, or a gym with your spouse is another enjoyable—and beneficial—way to spend time together. Some wellness centers have accessible pools and gym equipment that can be used by people with varying levels of physical ability, allowing you and your spouse to work out in the same facility. If you encourage your spouse to participate in exercise, swimming, or other sports with you, you will also benefit, by staying fit, reducing stress, and meeting other people who can provide social support and encouragement.

In addition to enhancing your relationship, social, physical, and recreational activities provide direct health benefits for the stroke survivor. Walking, bowling, gardening, and other physical activities promote physical recovery after stroke and confer psychological benefits such as improved mood and self-confidence. "Quiet times" like sharing a meal in a restaurant, watching a sunset, or sitting in a park are opportunities for emotional intimacy. And participating in activities that have social value—such as volunteering in a school or hospital, taking a class at a community or senior center, or becoming involved in local politics—can provide meaning, purpose, and identity for you and your spouse as individuals and as a couple.

Sometimes physical or cognitive impairments or depression will get in the way. Embarrassment and environmental barriers may create obstacles. As in other areas, you may need to negotiate with your spouse to get her involved in shared activities. Let your spouse know that it's essential to the health of your marriage to do things together for fun, that you have a need to continue your social life, and that her involvement—

both alone and with you—in social and recreational activities will improve her mood and promote her recovery. As part of the negotiation, you can offer to help your spouse conquer her fear or embarrassment. You can provide emotional support by exposing her only gradually to social situations or activities that make her anxious or uncomfortable and by helping her communicate more effectively with new people and handle negative reactions to her disability.

Advocating for your spouse can help him learn how to stand up for himself in social situations. For example, strangers in public or social situations (waiters, store clerks, and people you are meeting for the first time at a party) are likely to address their questions or conversation to you and ignore your spouse, especially if he uses a wheelchair or walker. It can be encouraging and instructive for your spouse to hear you ask the new person to please talk *directly to him*. You can help your spouse overcome embarrassment about having a disability or being "different" by discussing these feelings with him and trying out different ways for him to talk about his disability with others. Just as when you work to shape opportunities for your spouse to be more independent in self-care or household chores, you can make the effort to get your spouse participating in social activities. Doing so is an investment in your marriage that allows you to share a wider range of activities and experiences and to have more fun together. As your spouse improves, his interest in a variety of activities is likely to be rekindled— or he will find new interests—and he can gradually take a more active role in planning your shared social life.

Elaine has taken the lead in initiating and sustaining many of the hobbies and social activities that she and Stan have shared since his stroke. They both enjoy working on computer graphics and photography, but because of Stan's language impairments, Elaine has to help him get set up with a project and assist him if he has trouble navigating a particular computer program. Once Stan is "on a roll," they can both enjoy this activity, working either on the same project or on parallel projects. They have an active social life, frequently going to dinner with other couples, and they are involved with stroke organizations in their community. At first, Elaine scheduled all these social dates, but Stan now initiates plans with friends and makes decisions about where to eat or which movie to see. Although financial constraints prevent them from traveling as extensively as they would like, Elaine and Stan continue to take day trips and modest vacations. Now that Stan can drive, he makes a tangible contribution to their travels, giving Elaine a break to rest, plan their next sightseeing stop, or find a motel along their route.

Elaine also takes the lead in fostering their emotional intimacy. Although she feels that Stan's personality has changed since the stroke—he's more self-absorbed and less attuned to her needs—Elaine works hard to help Stan conquer his aphasia and to simplify their communication with each other, hoping this will encourage Stan to "tune in" more often. She uses humor and affection to bring out Stan's sense of fun, and she nurtures her role as his romantic partner. She also looks for creative ways to encourage Stan to share in and reciprocate her affection.

"We used to do more laughing and I miss that," she says. "Recently we were at the shore—we both love the water—and I said, 'See, we're having fun now. This is why I married you, because we love all the same things.' And he *got* that. Yesterday we were laughing, and it felt good. We always feel close, and I completely love him."

In a marriage that includes give and take by both spouses and a balance of caregiver–care recipient roles with partnership and emotional intimacy, the stage is set for a satisfying sexual relationship. Although the importance of sex varies from couple to couple, some degree of sexual intimacy and romance are essential in any good marriage. But many couples experience disruption of their love life after stroke, partly as a result of changes in body image, mood, and self-esteem that interfere with sexuality. Chapter 3 discusses the impact of stroke on romance and sexuality and explores how to maintain a satisfying sexual relationship with your spouse after stroke.

Practical Tips for Balancing the Roles of Caregiver and Marriage Partner

• Encourage your spouse's independence; start with small steps and add more responsibilities as your spouse improves.

- Be creative in finding ways that your spouse can contribute; get help from professionals if you need ideas.

- Don't expect your spouse to do every job perfectly; appreciate that she can do them well enough so that you don't have to.

- Get help with caregiving tasks, so you can focus on more enjoyable parts of your relationship.

- Try a variety of hobbies, social activities, and fun things to do with your spouse.

- Nurture the romance in your relationship—have dinner by candle-light, take a walk on the beach, have breakfast in bed.

CHAPTER 3

A Fine Romance

Sex and Intimacy after Stroke

Sex is very much on the minds of most stroke survivors and their spouses. You would think, then, that sexual function after stroke would receive its fair share of attention from the medical community. Unfortunately, though, among physicians and researchers, this topic has received far *less* attention than other aspects of stroke recovery. We hope this situation will change, because many stroke survivors are trying to cope with changes in their sexual function. Couples report that they have less interest in sex, are less satisfied with their sex lives, and have sexual intercourse less often after one partner has a stroke. In this chapter we discuss some of the common sexual problems after stroke and present some suggestions for improving your sexual relationship with your spouse.

If a person's sexual function changes after stroke, the change is almost certainly related to one or more of the following:

- the direct effects of the stroke on brain function,
- coexisting medical problems,
- side effects of medications,
- poor communication between partners, and
- psychological problems, such as depression or fear of sex.

The spouse of someone who has had a stroke is also affected by the stroke, in the sexual arena as well as in other areas of life. The spouse caregiver's depression, anxiety, and stress can lead to reduced sexual activity and satisfaction. Many other factors affect the sexual life of stroke survivors and their spouses, including attitudes about the importance of sex, comfort in discussing sex, willingness to participate in sex, self-esteem and self-image of both partners, role stress, and quality of the marital relationship. When it comes to sex after stroke, flexibility is an important factor: the partners' interest in and willingness to engage in a variety of techniques and approaches to sexual activity can be the key to sexual success.

As we saw in chapter 2, the role of caregiver can overwhelm other marital roles—friend, companion, romantic partner. This imbalance may have a negative effect on sexual intimacy. One crucial ingredient in recalibrating the marital relationship involves creating opportunities for the spouse with stroke to continue to make real contributions to the marriage. In other words, the marriage must continue to be a relationship of reciprocity, with both partners giving and taking. A couple's sexual relationship would seem to be a "natural" place for reciprocity to thrive—for stroke survivors and their spouses to both give and receive pleasure and to express mutual affection, love, and caring. But in reality, many couples find that resuming a satisfactory sexual relationship is the greatest challenge they face after stroke.

Physiological Problems with Sexual Function

A stroke can interfere with the body's ability to function sexually. A man may have difficulty getting or sustaining an erection, and a woman may not produce enough vaginal lubrication. These physiological problems can interfere with the "mechanics" of sex. Stroke survivors may also experience decreased sensation in some parts of the body, reducing their ability to become sexually aroused or to have an orgasm. Sexual function can be indirectly affected by other physical problems, too. If a person has bladder or bowel incontinence or has difficulty moving around in bed, the couple may not be able to use the sexual positions they enjoyed before the stroke. Either partner—or both—may have impaired sexual function because of other medical conditions, too, such as diabetes, hypertension, disorders of the prostate, or depression. Medications for treating high blood pressure, heart disease, depression, and other conditions can hamper a man's erectile function and decrease sexual desire, sexual excitement, and the ability to experience orgasm for both men and women.

Treating problems with sexual function can be difficult, especially when stroke-related impairments, other medical conditions, and side effects of medications are all involved.

Stan had experienced erectile dysfunction (ED) for several years before his stroke because of diabetes. He and his wife, Elaine, had enjoyed their sex life before the diabetes-related problem, and they experimented with various treatments for Stan's ED, including a penile pump that worked well. But after Stan's stroke, he could no longer use the pump on his own, because his right hand was weak. Elaine was afraid she would injure Stan if she helped him apply the pump, because, with his aphasia, he couldn't give her the guidance she needed. They still desired sexual intimacy and were pleased when one of their doctors suggested that Stan have a penile implant that would make erections possible. Elaine says this scares her, because Stan would have to go off Plavix to have the implant surgery (Plavix is a blood thinner that Stan takes to help prevent another stroke). They are currently weighing the risks and benefits of the implant procedure with Stan's primary-care doctor. Meanwhile, Elaine reports, "We cuddle . . . and we do what we can."

Elaine and Stan's experience illustrates two central points about sexual dysfunction after stroke:

- Discussing sexual dysfunction openly with a doctor who can recommend treatment options can be very helpful.
- Maintaining sexual intimacy and physical affection is important, even when sexual intercourse is not possible.

In fact, many of the physiological problems affecting sexual function can be treated effectively, if you and your spouse have a strong desire to maintain a good sexual relationship. Discussing sexual problems with your physician is a good place to start, not only for your spouse with stroke but also for yourself, if you are experiencing your own sexual difficulties related to medical problems, aging, or psychological stress. Some health care providers are uncomfortable talking about sex or will wrongly assume that you are not interested in sex or are not sexually active unless you raise the topic. You may not receive information and guidance about sexual activity until you ask for it.

A doctor can review your spouse's (and your) list of medications and identify which ones affect sexual function. The physician may be able to prescribe an alternative medication with fewer sexual side effects. Either your primary doctor or a specialist (such as a urologist or a gynecologist) may be able to suggest treatments for specific sexual problems, including medications, pumps, and implants for erectile dysfunction, and lubricants, hormone creams, and other treatments for reduced vaginal lubrication or decreased sexual desire. Your doctor may also be able to help you get better control of chronic medical conditions (like diabetes) that cause sexual dysfunction.

Doctors and nurses can also help you manage problems with bladder and bowel control to prevent accidents during sexual activity. There are simple solutions to several of these problems. It is a good practice to make sure the bladder or bowel is emptied before having sex and to limit drinking fluids for several hours before sex. Your spouse's doctor can help him regulate his bowel with medications, dietary routines, and bowel training programs so that bowel movements occur predictably at a certain time of the day. If your spouse uses a urinary catheter, it may be possible for you to remove it before having intercourse and reinsert it afterward. Or you can leave the catheter in place and cover it with a lubricated condom (for a man) or tape it to the abdomen (for a woman) during sexual intercourse. Your doctor or nurse can give you specific instructions about the safest way to manage your spouse's catheter during sex.

Finding a comfortable and effective position for sexual activity can be a challenge after a stroke, but if you are willing to experiment, a solution can probably be found. If your husband is unable to physically support himself in the man-on-top position (often called the "missionary" position) or cannot move his hips effectively to make thrusting motions, you may need to try alternative positions and take a more active role in sexual intercourse. To assist with positioning or make it more comfortable, try using multiple bed pillows or longer "body pillows." Some stroke survivors who have weakness on one side are afraid to lie on that side in bed. But if your spouse has weakness on one side, it is often better to lie on the weaker side during sex, so that the stronger side is free to move. This will allow your spouse to take a more active role in touching and foreplay. If pain or altered sensation causes discomfort during sex, try using sheets made of satin or soft cotton, which may reduce skin irritation.

If you and your spouse cannot find a comfortable position after trying these suggestions, your physician or a physical therapist may be able to help by working with your spouse to improve physical abilities such as flexibility, ability to move and change positions while in bed, endurance, range of motion in arms and legs, and fine motor coordination. Many couples become interested in resuming sexual activity after formal rehabilitation therapy services have ended. If your spouse is no longer working with a physical therapist, your doctor can refer her again. (Physical therapists generally provide treatment only after receiving a referral from a physician.) The doctor can specify on the referral the particular physical functions the therapist should work on to improve sexual function. Wanting to improve sexual function is a legitimate reason to see a physical therapist, and you should not feel reluctant to ask for this service if you need it.

Younger couples have concerns about issues of fertility and contraception. A stroke does not make a woman less fertile; a man's fertility is limited only if he has trouble ejaculating. (But if he does, this is definitely not a reliable method of birth control, since the problem can improve unexpectedly. Furthermore, a man can ejaculate even if he does not have a full erection or reach an orgasm during sex.) If the wife has not gone through menopause, the couple must continue to use contraception after stroke if pregnancy is not desired.

While many young people who have a stroke still want children and are able to raise them, pregnancy is medically risky for some women who have had a stroke; these risks should be discussed with your doctor *before* becoming pregnant. Birth control options should also be thoroughly explored with your doctor, since oral contraceptive pills may increase a woman's risk of having a second stroke. Other methods, such as a diaphragm or condom with spermicidal jelly or an intrauterine device (IUD), may be preferable after a stroke. If your spouse needs help inserting the diaphragm or putting on a condom, you can make such assistance a part of foreplay and sexual intimacy.

Although most stroke survivors and their spouses—including those who are incorrectly assumed to be too old for sex—have an interest in and questions about sexual function after stroke, these issues are often not adequately addressed by inpatient rehabilitation programs, and the topic is frequently skipped over by busy outpatient physicians. But if *you and your spouse* are willing to initiate a discussion of sex with your primary-care doctor or health care team, they will be able to help you or refer you to someone who can. If your doctor does not take your sexual concerns seriously, you should ask for a referral to someone who is better qualified. Helpful information on sex and stroke is available from books, stroke organizations, and Internet sites (see the Resources section in this book).

Psychosocial Issues

Sexual dysfunction that results directly from a stroke (not from medications or other medical problems) will likely improve over time; it is *not* the major cause of sexual problems for people recovering from a stroke. In most cases, psychological and emotional factors are responsible for the difficulty in sexual adjustment experienced by stroke survivors and their spouses.

Fear of Another Stroke

Craig's stroke was due to bleeding from a vascular malformation in his brain. After he had surgery to repair the malformation, Craig's doctor told them that sex would most likely be safe, but he and his wife, Laura, were so afraid of causing another bleed that they waited two years, until Craig's brain scan was completely "clean," before resuming sexual intercourse.

While there is little evidence that sexual activity will cause another stroke, it is a good idea to get reassurance on this matter by asking your spouse's doctor whether he can safely engage in sexual intercourse. If you are afraid that sexual activity will put too much physical stress on your spouse's heart, then ask the doctor about that specifically, and about whether he should take a less strenuous position (for example, lying down on his back or side, or sitting during sex).

Uneasiness about "Experimenting"

Most couples develop a regular sexual routine and are comfortable with a particular range of sexual practices. For some couples, sexual intimacy always includes intercourse, while for others, oral sex or other forms of sexual contact may be acceptable variations. After a stroke, your spouse may have difficulty participating in intercourse because of one or more of the physiological problems discussed above. If you think you have "failed" at sex because of this, you may be reluctant to try again, and your sex life can evaporate. But if you are willing to try different types of sexual activity that are less dependent on "performance," then both of you can continue to experience sensual pleasure and sexual satisfaction. It may be helpful to think about starting your sex life over, as if you were teenagers—beginning with kissing, "petting," and mutual masturbation. The use of sex toys, vibrators, watching erotic movies, or giving your spouse a sensuous massage may enhance your sexual excitement. If you haven't had oral sex with your spouse before her stroke, you can try adding it to your repertoire. Whatever you do, try to suspend your judgment about being "successful" or having sex the "right" way, and focus instead on enjoying closeness and creating pleasure for yourself and your spouse.

Communicating about Sex

Some spouses believe that sexual activity is appropriate only for healthy people. They are afraid that after a stroke it will be psychologically damaging for the stroke survivor. This is rarely the case—most people retain an interest in sex after stroke and are capable of sexual pleasure. Your spouse may be hesitant to initiate sexual activity for various reasons. She may feel less attractive than before the stroke or be worried about disappointing you because of changes in her mobility or other functions affecting sexual performance. You can help by initiating a discussion of sexual concerns and desires and by confirming that you are interested in resuming a sexual relationship with her.

In fact, *communication* about sexual matters is an essential ingredient of sexual success for couples after stroke (just as it is for other couples). Those couples who do not discuss sex with one another after a stroke experience more dissatisfaction with their sex lives and have less frequent sexual relations. Communication not only confirms your mutual interest in sex but creates the opportunity for you and your spouse to discuss and begin solving problems that may be preventing a satisfactory sex life. Sometimes communication about sex is hindered by cognitive or language impairments related to stroke, such as aphasia; this topic is discussed in more detail below.

Depression

Depression, too, can play a role in reducing sexual satisfaction after stroke. Depression can weaken a person's interest in sex, hamper sexual performance (such as maintaining erection or lubrication), and directly impair the ability to enjoy sexual activity. Because depression is common in both stroke survivors and caregivers after a stroke, the possibility of depression should be considered whenever interest or pleasure in sex seems lacking. Treatment with antidepressant medications or psychotherapy, or both, often leads to greater interest in sex and increased sexual pleasure. Some antidepressant medications contribute to sexual problems such as ED or difficulty experiencing an orgasm, but not everyone has these side effects. Your doctor can choose a medication with less chance of these effects if she or he knows that sex is a priority for you. For some people who do experience minor side effects from antidepressant medication, these are outweighed by the improvement in mood, energy, and interest in sex.

Aphasia

Communication problems posed by speech and language deficits present a special set of challenges to sexual functioning after stroke. Aphasia may make it difficult for couples to discuss the emotional nuances of sex, to communicate specific sexual desires or affection to each other, or even to let each other know whether sexual contact is wanted. Although sex can be largely nonverbal, many couples use talking before and during sex to enhance their sexual pleasure. It may feel strange to initiate sex without talking about it, and some readjustment may be required to engage in sex without being able to use speech to share fantasies, express pleasure or displeasure, or send other sexual signals.

Eli and Janet are generally optimistic, creative, and persistent people, and they have coped exceptionally well with Eli's aphasia, which was the major lasting effect of his stroke. Over the three years since his stroke, Eli's language skills have improved, and he has taken on more responsibilities in the marriage—doing most of the housework, cooking, and carpooling their teenagers, while Janet works outside the home. Janet reports that the most challenging aspect of their life after stroke is that their "intimacy as a couple is different now. We're at a new in-between phase [in communication ability]." Eli jokes that before he regained the ability to talk, they had "nonverbal sex . . . like animals." Now that he can communicate basic information but continues to have difficulty conveying subtle and complex feelings, Janet finds herself more dissatisfied with their sex life. The lack of verbal communication seems to be more difficult now, in part because her expectations have increased. She notes that Eli has done so well, she is surprised and disappointed when his limitations come to the foreground.

Couples like Eli and Janet may benefit from taking a step back and considering where they were before their sex life stalled—in this case, Eli and Janet had "nonverbal" sex, which was comfortable and enjoyable in the early phases of recovery. By focusing on nonverbal aspects of sex and sexual communication, couples can reduce their focus on speech—if the stroke survivor's limitations are disappointing and frustrating—and concentrate instead on enhancing their pleasure through nonverbal means. Verbal communication during sex can then be gradually reintroduced as speech and language abilities improve. Experimenting with different types of talking to see what enhances or detracts from mutual pleasure is the next step.

If your spouse has expressive aphasia, she may need to use more overt physical signals during sexual encounters. These include pointing to or placing your hand on the place she wants to be touched, or pantomiming sexual acts or movements. If your spouse has trouble understanding complex speech, it may also be necessary for you to communicate your desires to him in a similar nonverbal fashion. Before the stroke, you may not have used physical gestures in this way, and it might feel awkward at first. But as with other areas of adaptation after stroke, keeping an open mind and experimenting with a variety of communication techniques can lead to improvement in intimacy.

You can also create a setting that enhances the mood for sex by using romantic music and lighting, and you can share preparations for sexual activity, such as taking a shower together, to add to the success of nonverbal (or verbal) sexual experiences. Including verbal communication in your sexual encounters may be more or less possible, depending on the extent of your spouse's aphasia, but an attitude of experimentation without set expectations for the success of verbal communications will help avoid disappointment and frustration. Many people who have aphasia can hear the "music" behind the words—they are able to comprehend the emotional tones or meanings of speech. So your spouse may respond positively to your verbal expressions of love, desire, approval, or pleasure, even if she does not understand every word. Using a combination of touch, gesture, facial expression, and talking can improve your intimate connection with your spouse who has communication problems; these approaches can be helpful for any couple experiencing problems with intimacy after a stroke.

Cognitive Deficits

Limitations of memory, reasoning ability, or judgment may also interfere with sexual intimacy after a stroke. Cognitive problems that cause poor control of impulses, limit one's ability to initiate activities, or make it difficult to create new memories can give the impression that the stroke survivor has become "a different person," and such feelings can affect both emotional and sexual intimacy. Some spouse caregivers feel less sexually attracted to a stroke survivor whose cognitive disabilities result in more "childish" behaviors, such as ignoring social conventions, showing poor judgment, or requiring frequent repetition to learn simple information. These behaviors can affect sexuality by altering the stroke survivor's self-presentation or personal appearance.

Mike and Doris have some disagreements about whether Doris is "dressed properly." Since her right-brain stroke, she is less aware of her appearance and sometimes dresses in ways that Mike considers inappropriate. He notes that "she can't put on her bra" but that "she doesn't care; she'll go without it," so he puts it on for her. Sometimes she doesn't get her pants pulled up all the way in the back, and although it doesn't seem to matter to Doris, Mike pulls up her pants so she won't be "exposed." Doris says she and Mike are "basically mellow people," and they are able to negotiate this and other aspects of their marriage without much conflict. Although Mike is uncomfortable with Doris's reduced concern for her appearance, his ability to express his discomfort, his offers to help, and her willingness to defer to his judgment on this issue have prevented it from becoming a major turnoff. In fact, he and Doris have been able to discuss and plan for sexual intimacy: "Like we'll say 'Tonight's the night.'" They have times when sexual contact is less frequent, but they agree that "when it's going, it's going well."

A satisfactory sexual relationship may also be disrupted if your spouse has severe memory problems and can't remember when or how frequently you have had sex. Sometimes this can cause your spouse to lose interest in sex or to want to have sex more often than you desire.

For Beth and Wayne, sexual intimacy seems to be the "last frontier" of marital adjustment after his stroke. Wayne's severe difficulty with memory makes it hard for him to engage in solving the problem: he knows that their sex life is different, but he can't remember why or how it changed. "We're not as active as we once were. I guess that's all because of me. I don't really know . . . maybe it's because we're getting older." Beth says the problem is lack of any sexual relationship. She recalls that their sex life had "lessened to nothing" *before* the stroke, probably for multiple reasons, including Wayne's medications, stress, and some marital tensions. Beth says she would like to rekindle their sex life, but the problem now is that "he doesn't even think about it," and when she brings it up, "he can't remember what happened before, so we can't really go back and try to figure it out." Beth gets frustrated with the fact that sex is yet another area where she needs to initiate every discussion, provide reminders of past conversations, and take the lead if she and Wayne are to move forward with their sexual relationship. Even when she does try to initiate lovemaking, Wayne is not always receptive to her approach. "My efforts are too assertive and he doesn't like that—and his efforts are none!"

If your situation is like Beth and Wayne's, there are several strategies that can help. You can communicate about sex, and resume sexual contact, by using the same mental and behavioral strategies that you might apply to other areas of your spouse's functioning that are affected by memory or cognitive problems. For example, you can begin to have regular discussions with your spouse about your sexual relationship, make notes during each discussion (and review them together before the next one), use a calendar or diary to chart when sexual intimacy or intercourse has taken place, and schedule times for sexual intimacy in the weekly routine.

If your spouse has trouble remembering the history of sexual problems in your marriage, it might be helpful to reconstruct a simple timeline for her, so that she can better understand what has happened in your relationship and why you feel the way you do. You will probably need to write this down, so she can refer to it as needed. However, focusing on the past may not be particularly constructive if your spouse's memory for events before the stroke is very poor. It might make more sense to start with discussing what is going on in your relationship *now*, and enlist your spouse's support in planning to change your relationship (for example, to have sex more often or less often), taking into account what each of you desires. For some people, getting marriage therapy from a psychologist or sex therapist who understands both the cognitive consequences of stroke and the dynamics of intimate relationships is helpful.

If your spouse lacks sexual initiative because of cognitive impairment, you may feel awkward about asking for sexual contact. While your spouse may passively acquiesce to your sexual overtures, his failure to initiate, his lack of enthusiasm, or his reduced emotional responsiveness may lead you to feel that you are "taking advantage of" or coercing him. In this situation, you may feel more comfortable initiating sexual contact in incremental stages, starting with kissing, hugging, and caressing. Once you feel assured that your partner is comfortable with the experience, you can gradually add other sexual activities. Remember to communicate with your partner, asking whether he wants to continue and what type of sexual touching feels good to him. It may be helpful not to have sexual intercourse as your goal for a time, but to focus instead on creating a comfortable, relaxed, and pleasurable experience, to spark your spouse's interest in sexual contact.

Loss of Desire for Sex

To find solutions to problems in your sex life after a stroke, both you *and* your spouse must want to resume your sexual relationship—and most couples do want this. Rarely, though, a stroke survivor loses all desire for sex, is unwilling or unable to make the necessary adjustments, or flat-out refuses to participate in a sexual relationship. This can happen when a person has stroke-related dementia or personality changes, debilitating medical illnesses, or serious psychiatric problems.

A caregiver spouse may find it impossible—or unhealthy—to remain in a marriage where she handles all the household responsibilities, makes all the major decisions, provides numerous hours of caregiving, *and* is deprived of sexual gratification. But divorce may not be feasible economically or practically, and it could leave the stroke survivor without adequate care or resources. A caregiver may *want* to provide physical care, supervision, emotional support, and companionship for his spouse—provided his sexual needs can be met elsewhere.

Some caregivers arrange an informal "sexual contract" with a friend—agreeing to have periodic sexual relations without further emotional involvement or commitment—while continuing to live with and care for their spouse. A stroke survivor who has no interest in sex may consent to such an arrangement; but a caregiver can reasonably make this decision on his own if his spouse is unable to understand the problem or negotiate a solution. For many people, sex outside of marriage is intolerable on moral, religious, or legal grounds or is emotionally challenging because it separates sex from love. But in some instances, finding sexual gratification outside the marriage allows a caregiver to *remain* in the marriage—and to continue providing love, support, and care for her spouse.

Hypersexuality

Occasionally a stroke survivor—usually after a stroke affecting the thalamus or temporal lobe brain areas—is unable to inhibit or control sexual impulses, resulting in *hypersexuality* (inappropriate and excessive overtly sexual behavior). He may want to have sex very frequently or at inappropriate times, such as when the grandchildren are visiting, or he may attempt to initiate sex by making obscene remarks, physically grabbing you, or exposing himself. These behaviors tend to be a sexual turnoff and may be frightening. You can try to instruct your spouse in the use of subtler, more appropriate ways to signal her interest in sex, but this approach may or may not be effective. You may be able to re-direct her attention by offering an alternative activity or distraction. If you are not interested in sex and your spouse seems unable to inhibit his desire, you can try pointing him to a private place where he can masturbate. Your spouse may also make inappropriate sexual advances to health care providers, friends, relatives, or even strangers. If she be-comes inappropriately sexual in public or her hypersexuality leads to agitation or aggression, you should seek help from a physician with expertise in neurobehavioral syndromes who will be able to prescribe medications and give you further advice on behavioral management.

Changes in Roles and Self-Image

Resuming an enjoyable sex life can be difficult for a caregiver who pro-vides frequent hands-on care and regularly helps her spouse with ac-tivities of daily living, such as bathing, going to the toilet, dressing, eating, or transferring from bed to chair. If you provide extensive per-sonal care for your spouse, you may begin to feel like his nurse or par-ent rather than his wife. Some caregiver spouses find it hard to shed this role and slip back into the role of romantic and sexual partner. Caregivers may be "turned off" by having to help their partners with toileting or personal hygiene, and stroke survivors may feel embarrassed or ashamed about needing this type of care from their partners.

Caregivers who do not provide personal care for their spouses, but who take on many additional responsibilities to keep their home and marriage functioning after their partner's stroke, may also experience significant role changes that affect their self-image and their view of their partner—and thus their sexual relationship. After Stan's stroke, for example, Elaine took care of him 24 hours a day. Rarely were they apart for more than a few hours. As she took on more responsibilities for the finances and decision making and started working part time, she found herself becoming impatient with Stan, and now she was wor-ried about things that Stan used to handle.

"Stan doesn't have to worry like I do now. We have no security really. I'm working because it pays for food and entertainment. Stan doesn't get it, he can't see the big picture [of our finances]. It's hard to get mad at him, but I do, more than I used to. I think it's because I've had a taste of being on my own at work. [Before the stroke] I was the clinging vine. I worshiped the man, and just expected him to do everything. But now I do everything. And he's become so dependent on me. I've never fallen out of love with him, [but] he's a different person now."

Elaine experienced a role reversal in her relationship with Stan. Since the stroke, she has taken on many of the roles that Stan previously had in their marriage—breadwinner, financial manager, and social planner. While she perceives Stan as being a "different person," she clearly feels different, too; no longer the "clinging vine," she is now the primary decision maker and director of their relationship.

For some caregiving spouses, this type of role reversal changes their sense of themselves as "feminine" or "masculine," making them feel less sexy or attractive. These role changes can also make your partner less attractive to you—because of his need for personal care or his dependence, you may view him as less "manly," even though you continue to love him deeply. Just talking to your spouse may be all that's needed to restore a positive image of yourself and your spouse and to renew your interest in a sexual relationship. If you find that talking to your spouse is difficult or is not helping, then professional counseling can help you incorporate your changed marital roles into a new self-image, allowing you to reexperience yourself as an attractive (and interested) sexual partner.

If aphasia makes verbal communication difficult, as in Stan's case, it may be more helpful for you to work on relieving the stress about your changing role by getting more social support and respite care, or paying more attention to activities that enhance your own sexual self-image and interest (such as exercise, spa treatments, massage, and the like). You may want to "set the stage" for sexual activity by helping your partner to look or behave in ways that are more attractive to you. In these situations you may benefit from creating a more romantic environment to enhance sexual expression, such as dressing up for a date, wearing sexy clothing or lingerie, using dim lighting or candles and playing romantic music in the bedroom, getting away for a weekend at a hotel, or anything else that you find conducive to intimacy.

Time Management and Fatigue

Time management and fatigue also put a damper on sexual activity after a stroke. In the early stages of recovery, fatigue can be debilitating for stroke survivors, but even months or years later, a survivor may become fatigued more rapidly than before the stroke. Fatigue causes a decline in functions of all kinds. You as the caregiver may also experience fatigue, especially if you are providing full-time care or are combining caregiving with other responsibilities such as work or raising children. Often, both spouses are physically and emotionally depleted by the end of the day.

> Beth and Wayne tried taking a trip without their children, thinking it would stimulate romance. But they also tried to squeeze in an afternoon of sightseeing, without realizing how exhausting that would be. After dinner at a nice restaurant, they went back to the hotel, watched TV, and went to sleep. Beth says she is "always fatigued; there's always something to be done." Improving their sex life seems to take a backseat to other tasks. "I have so many things on my plate that I can't get to that," she says.

Because fatigue can be a major hindrance to resuming your sexual relationship after stroke, it is essential to make sexual intimacy a priority and to set aside enough time and energy to increase your chance of a pleasurable experience. Before your spouse's stroke, you might have been able to have sex at the end of a full day, but that may not work for you now. "Bedtime" is not generally the best time for sex after a stroke; sexual experiences will likely be more satisfying for you and your spouse if both of you are adequately rested and not pressed for time. The best time for sex might be in the late morning or in the early afternoon after a nap. For stroke survivors or for caregivers who are working or have strenuous routines, sexual intimacy may best be scheduled for a weekend when there are no other commitments.

Scheduling sex may seem unromantic, or you may worry that lack of spontaneity will affect the "mood" for sex. But scheduling sex can be seen as an acknowledgment that sex is a high priority for your relationship; it signifies a commitment to each other. Once couples get used to the idea of scheduling sex, they may begin to enjoy the anticipation of a romantic encounter. If you feel guilty about making sex a priority, and if setting aside time for sex in the middle of the day feels "decadent," remember that sex, like walking and cooking, is an activity of daily living that is affected by stroke; practicing new ways of "doing it" is part of recovery. Having sex is at least as vital to your spouse's sense of well-being as receiving physical therapy for walking, and can be enjoyable for you as well as your partner.

Use It Before You Lose It

Sexual function after stroke is similar to other aspects of physical and social function: it may not be perfect, and it may not be the same as it was before the stroke, but repeated practice is likely to bring improvement. Despite limitations, it can still be immensely enjoyable. Think of the old saying, "It's not what you've got, but what you *do* with what you've got!" Although adaptations may be required, your reinvigorated sexual relationship can be a source of pleasure and can make you feel fulfilled and close to your spouse.

> Craig reports that once he and Laura were ready to resume having sex, he needed "some assistance" in the form of medication to help sustain his erections. "I would like it if I were less reliant on artificial stimuli. I'd rather go back to the way it was, but you can't go back there. You've got to accept what is and move on. Unfortunately, most insurance companies and drug plans don't pay for erectile dysfunction medication. It's very expensive stuff—so you use it judiciously!"

You might find, like Craig and Laura, that the need to use ED medication "judiciously" is another good reason to carefully plan and prioritize sexual activity and avoid letting your sex life be derailed by fatigue or other distractions.

For you and your spouse, accepting changes in his or her body and being willing to move ahead with new ways of participating are key elements in maintaining sexual function and a good sexual relationship.

The three essential ingredients for resuming a satisfactory sex life after stroke are *desire* (wanting to resume sexual activity), *communication* (verbal or nonverbal), and *opportunity* (making the time for sex). With these ingredients in place, you can experiment with a variety of ways to give and receive sensual pleasure. Sexual intimacy need not always include sexual intercourse; if erectile or other physical problems make intercourse impossible, other forms of sexual expression can be gratifying. Kissing and cuddling, massage, oral sex, mutual masturbation, and use of sex toys or vibrators are some of the activities you can enjoy even if intercourse is not an option.

Like other areas of function after a stroke, recovery of sexual function and sexual satisfaction do not happen overnight. Resuming an active sex life takes patience, practice, and a positive attitude. Efforts to revive a sex life that is waning after a stroke will be rewarded with great pleasure and satisfaction for both you and your spouse and may provide additional benefits such as improving your spouse's muscle strength and endurance and elevating both your and your spouse's moods.

Practical Tips for Sex and Intimacy after Stroke

- Talk to your spouse about your sexual relationship. Make it a high priority, not the last thing on your list.

- Talk with your spouse's doctor about whether your spouse is able to safely engage in sexual intercourse, and ask for help with sexual problems related to stroke, medications, other medical conditions, or depression.

- Ask the doctor for specific instructions on managing your spouse's urinary catheter during sex.

- If your spouse wants help with sustaining an erection, ask his doctor about treatments, including medications, pumps, and penile implants.

- Use water-based vaginal lubricants for increased comfort during sex.

- If you or your spouse is depressed, get treatment with medication or psychotherapy or both.

- Experiment with a variety of sexual activities, such as kissing, petting, and oral sex; focus on pleasure and intimacy, not "performance."

- Try different positions to improve sexual pleasure and increase your spouse's comfort; use pillows for extra support.

- If your spouse has aphasia, both of you can use gestures, facial expression, and touch to communicate your sexual desires.

- Have sex when you and your spouse are well rested and have plenty of time.

- Encourage your spouse to keep up her personal hygiene and dress in ways that you find attractive.

- Avoid becoming overloaded with caregiving responsibilities. You will feel sexier if you take care of yourself and do things that make you feel attractive.

- If your spouse has an impaired memory, try using a calendar to keep track of when you have had sex, and make a schedule for sexual activity.

- If your spouse has cognitive problems that interfere with initiating sex, you can take the lead; start slowly and make sure your spouse is agreeable before going further.

- If you need additional help with sexual issues after a stroke, consider seeing a marriage therapist or a sex therapist familiar with stroke. The American Association of Sexuality Educators, Counselors, and Therapists can help you find a therapist who understands disability and stroke issues. This organization can be found at www .aasect.org.

CHAPTER 4

Give Me a Break

Support for the Caregiving Spouse

It's pretty clear that strong relationships are built when both partners contribute to the relationship and share mutually enjoyable activities. But most couples also need to socialize, relax, and be supported outside the relationship as well as within it. Indeed, few marriages—even the best of them—meet all the needs of both spouses. Most people need an occasional "break" from their spouse to pursue their own friendships and hobbies, read, take a walk, or just quietly reflect on life.

Having the opportunity to "recharge your batteries," whether alone or with friends and family, is even more important when you are a caregiving spouse, especially if you are overloaded with heavy care demands or if you are providing care and also performing multiple other roles. As a caregiver, you have to make time to care for *yourself*—both to keep yourself healthy (physically and mentally) and to manage stress. You can take care of yourself by getting social support, from friends and family or by using community services; attending to your medical and mental health care needs; and learning to be your own advocate.

Social Support for Caregivers

Earlier we talked about how social support for the stroke survivor improves his general health and optimizes his recovery from a stroke. But social support is beneficial for *you* as well as for your spouse. Social support for caregivers improves their mood, reduces their stress, and increases their satisfaction with life.

Social support comes in many forms. Instrumental, or practical, support includes help with practical tasks as well as access to information, education, or training that makes caregiving easier. Emotional support includes empathy, affection, friendship, and sharing of feelings, ideas, and enjoyable activities. Both types of support are valuable for caregivers. Practical support reduces the physical and time demands of caregiving or makes caregivers more confident and efficient, and sometimes both. Emotional support counteracts the stress of caregiving by providing positive and pleasurable emotional experiences and feelings and perhaps by changing one's negative view of life circumstances to a more positive view. Both types of social support for caregivers are available from family, friends, community sources, and health care providers.

Asking for Help—and Accepting It

To gain the benefits of social support, you have to accept the idea that it's okay to ask others for help. "Taking care of yourself" is not just an abstract idea; it means changing your behavior—and enlisting or allowing others to support you by helping with caregiving tasks or in other ways.

> People are always saying to me, "Don't forget to take care of yourself." And I swear, if I hear that one more time, I'll scream! I don't have time to take care of myself. If they're so concerned about it, why don't they offer to *do* something? Why don't they say, "I'll take Jim to his therapy this week—or I'll sit with Jim while you go out for awhile"?—Mary, caregiver for her husband Jim.

Like Mary, many caregivers, especially in the early months after their spouse's stroke, feel overwhelmed by the demands and stresses of caregiving and are unable to get away. Their friends and family may not spontaneously offer to help. The natural reaction is to feel unsupported and angry. When offers of help are not forthcoming, though, you have to *ask* for help. A well-defined request for help will often produce a positive response: ask specifically about getting a ride, having someone stay with your spouse for two hours, or having a neighbor pick up a few groceries for you. In most cases, family and friends do offer to help, and then the challenge for caregivers is learning to accept with grace and gratitude.

One recent interview study concluded that "the work of caregiving is nearly impossible to maintain without the social support of family and friends in the community." Yet this study also noted that, even when they knew family members were willing to help, caregivers were hesitant to call on them for regular assistance. Mike has had the experience of knowing he needs help and being uncomfortable with asking for it.

> "Men are reluctant to ask for help, but a lot of people will offer it. They *want* to help you." Mike acknowledges that he hasn't been away from Doris for more than four hours at a stretch in the past three years and that in some situations it would be better for Doris to have help from a woman—such as taking her shopping for clothes. Instead, Mike has "had to learn to deal with embarrassment" when he takes Doris into fitting rooms or restrooms at department stores. He knows that there are friends and family who would be happy to help, but, he says, "I can't ask for help."

An unwillingness to ask for help—or to accept it—may reflect a concern that you will lose the sense of independence or privacy as a couple that you previously enjoyed. Having an "outsider" help with your spouse's care can feel like an invasion of your "marital space." You may also feel that sharing your needs and problems with another person is a betrayal of your spousal loyalty, or that by accepting help you are shirking your duty as a spouse.

Guilt feelings can be intensified if your spouse insists that you are the *only* person he wants to provide his care, and if he actively resists being helped by anyone else. This is a common source of conflict between spouses. You can resolve the dilemma best if you keep in mind that your spouse may also be trying to protect his privacy and the special relationship you have with each other. He may be afraid that other caregivers will not be as competent or empathic as you, or he may simply be so preoccupied with his own needs and difficulties that he has lost perspective on how caregiving affects your life. It can be helpful to talk with your spouse about *your* need for help and to remind him that accepting help from someone else will be helpful for both of you.

You can help your spouse understand that having others help with caregiving does not mean you are abandoning her or that you care less about her. You can also negotiate with your spouse about the type of help she feels more comfortable accepting from another person (such as getting rides or help with cooking versus assistance with dressing or bathing) and about the best time of the day or week for you to take a break. Your spouse also may be more accepting of outside help if it enables him to do things he enjoys and which you might not be able to do (or don't enjoy doing) with him, such as attending a men's club event at church, having lunch with his best friend, shopping and trying on clothes, or watching a football game on TV. If you present the idea that a break from caregiving for you is also an opportunity for him to increase his own enjoyment, he will be more likely to see it as a win-win situation.

Aside from guilt feelings, you might hesitate to ask for help because you fear becoming a burden to others or don't want to feel beholden to them. But, as Mike pointed out, people often *want* to help, and giving help can be very rewarding for the giver as well as the recipient. However, even when people want to help, they will tend to back off if their initial offers are rejected. Discussing your concerns and feelings with potential helpers might improve your understanding of why they want to help, reassure you that they are not expecting any "payback," and keep their offers coming. Ultimately, you have a responsibility to yourself and your spouse to be receptive to offers of help, to say "Yes, please!" when someone asks if you want help. The more you ask for help and allow others to help, the more you will build your confidence about accepting assistance.

Some caregivers find it easier to accept practical support from their community network than from close family members. Practical social support can come from people who are not necessarily close friends, such as volunteers from religious organizations, schools, community groups, or neighbors. Berenice Kleiman, who wrote a book about caring for her husband after his stroke, gives this advice: "You can't do everything on your own, especially at the beginning. If friends aren't available, seek out a volunteer group that provides such help, perhaps your municipality, county, church, or synagogue. You'll need help to pick up medications, prepare healthy meals, or even cover for you as you step away for a few minutes [of personal time]." This sentiment is echoed repeatedly by experienced caregivers and by health care providers who work with caregivers. "Let family and friends help. . . . Give them a chance. . . . You have to reach out for help and you have to ask for help from anyone you can."

Practical support can involve working directly with your spouse in tasks such as bathing or transporting her, or it can be more general help with household tasks such as shopping, cleaning, or cooking that free up your time to attend to your own health, social, or relaxation needs.

> After Luis's stroke, Toni had help from his mother, who stayed with them for several months. Her assistance with the day-to-day tasks of caregiving left Toni with more time to work, pay attention to the children, and exercise. In addition, Toni's friends frequently brought meals for the family. One friend even offered to pay for a house-cleaning service. Toni notes that she had "read a pamphlet about taking care of the caregiver" while Luis was in rehab—and she took it to heart. Her advice: "I tell other caregivers not to feel guilty about taking time for themselves."

As Marty Richards points out in her book *Caresharing,* caregiver "independence" is a myth. People need each other, and the normal state of affairs for human beings is *inter*dependence—we are all both givers and receivers of help and support. She likens the process of caregiving to a "dance where you move back and forth to the rhythms you sense for yourself and the one receiving your care. It is a dance with multiple partners, including caregivers and care receivers alike, friends and family, the community of faith, and healthcare professionals."

In seeking and accepting help from your extended family or community networks, remember that those who assist and support you with caregiving will also reap benefits from the experience. Family and friends who are close to you and your spouse likely want to be involved in the work of caregiving, and helping out gives them opportunities to be emotionally close and to share the enjoyment and the satisfaction of making a contribution to your spouse's recovery. Many people find that giving help to others is a deeply satisfying expression of love or a pathway to enhancing their personal or spiritual growth. Others may have special talents for or interests in cooking, home repairs, driving, reading, and so forth that they are eager to share with you and your spouse not only because you need these things but because they enjoy doing them. Sharing the experience of caregiving can be a positive experience for everyone involved.

Respite Care

Respite care is a particular kind of support for caregivers. Basically, *respite* means a break! Respite care allows the caregiver to take a break from caregiving while someone else takes over temporarily. Although any break from caregiving, even for an hour, could be called a respite, the term is generally used for periods of several hours scheduled regularly, or sometimes for longer breaks that allow the full-time caregiver to take a vacation, get away for a weekend, pursue a work or home project, or attend to her own medical care.

Respite care is particularly important if you are providing 24-hour care for your spouse and cannot leave him alone because of cognitive or communication impairments, severe mobility impairments, or unsafe behavior. Sometimes it is difficult to find a family member or friend to provide respite care for a stroke survivor with severe disability or dementia. In such situations, respite care can be provided by trained professionals: nursing assistants (or nurses, if needed) who can be found through home health agencies or privately, through newspaper ads and recommendations from other families. Nurses or certified nursing assistants (CNAs) can be hired to provide respite care in your own home in the daytime or overnight.

Adult day care facilities or senior citizen center programs may be appropriate for your spouse. These facilities and programs allow caregivers to get a break for one or more days during the week. Centers for adult day care (sometimes referred to as medical day care or senior day care) may be affiliated with hospitals or rehabilitation facilities, or they may be freestanding facilities in the community. These centers provide supervision, medication management, meals, stimulating activities such as crafts, music, classes, and community outings, and sometimes physical, occupational, or speech therapy services. Some facilities provide transportation. Most are available for as many week-days per week as needed.

If you are going away for a week or more, you might look into re-spite care in a respite care center or nursing home, where your spouse can stay overnight. This is a reasonable alternative to hiring an indi-vidual nurse or nursing assistant to stay in your home, and it may be more affordable. Respite care in a nursing home setting allows you to attend to necessary business or take time for a pleasure trip or a good rest, with the knowledge that your spouse is getting appropriate medi-cal care in a safe and supervised environment. Most people who go to a nursing home today stay for a limited period of time, generally no longer than a few weeks. Nursing homes no longer carry the old stigma of "putting your relative away and throwing away the key."

Some facilities offer respite weekends, which may include recre-ational and other enrichment experiences for your spouse to enjoy while you are getting a break. You may be able to find such programs through the local stroke association or your local government's office on disability or aging.

Emotional Support

Emotional support from your friends, family members, or religious or community organizations is essential. It can enable you to cope with stress and provide positive emotional experiences that enhance your sense of well-being. Emotional support can prevent depression for you and promote feelings of optimism and hopefulness. Many spouse caregivers find they need to develop new social networks or substan-tially enhance existing relationships with friends and family to coun-ter the emotional isolation that may set in after their spouse has a stroke. Seeking out emotional support will likely help you cope better with the stresses and strains of caregiving and give you emotional en-ergy that you can bring back into your marriage.

Friends and relatives are the most common sources for emotional support. The opportunity to regularly talk and share feelings with an understanding listener can help you emotionally, even if this contact is over the phone. Rita, for example, has a good friend from out of town who calls her every night. She feels it's essential to "share what you're going through. The more you keep something inside you, it just festers." Sharing with her friend each night gives Rita the chance to unburden herself of whatever problems she may have faced that day. Beth, who goes out regularly with her women friends, finds that having fun with them boosts her spirits. Although Toni's extended family lives out of state, she finds emotional support from friends, co-workers, and her husband's family that is valuable in helping her cope. Says Toni, "I think that we were so lucky because of our family and friends. At the beginning, I didn't have much contact with friends, but now I do."

Family and friends can listen with empathy, offer comfort in times of loss, share enjoyable activities, laugh and joke with you, or express affection, and they can help you solve problems by sharing their ideas and perspectives. They can offer validation and reinforcement, boosting your confidence in yourself. But sometimes, family and friends lack the knowledge base to help you cope with complex emotional and social problems related to stroke and its consequences. Many spouses find that stroke clubs or support groups fill an important role in providing support that is specifically tailored to their experiences as caregivers.

Stroke Clubs

Stroke clubs are support groups for stroke survivors and their family caregivers. These groups are sponsored by national, state, or county stroke associations and generally meet at hospitals, assisted living centers, senior centers, or other community facilities. You can find a stroke club in your area through the National Stroke Association or the American Stroke Association (see contact information in the Resources section of this book). Stroke clubs usually combine social support and education. A typical meeting features a professional speaker on some aspect of stroke, followed by a social hour.

Some clubs have separate groups just for caregivers, while at others caregivers and stroke survivors attend together. Many states have stroke clubs or stroke support groups that focus on particular subgroups, such as young stroke survivors, stroke survivors with aphasia, or spouse or family caregivers. Support groups specifically for caregivers can also be found through local hospitals and senior centers. Such groups often include caregivers of people with various diagnoses. You may want to "audit" a few groups to find the one most compatible with your needs.

Attending a stroke club or support group for caregivers is an excellent way to find people who share your experience. Many caregivers (and stroke survivors) develop lasting and mutually supportive friendships with people they meet at these groups. Rita, whose social life is limited, finds much solace in her monthly caregiver support group meetings. She also attends a stroke club with her husband. These groups help her stay "upbeat" and put her problems in perspective by letting her see that she is "not the worst off." Mike, despite his difficulty in asking friends and family for help, has benefited from the support of a stroke club. He found it important as a source of both emotional support and practical information. "When Doris first had the stroke," Mike explains, "I had an empty feeling in my head. There were so many issues to resolve. The stroke club is social, plus you get ideas. You find out you're not alone, and you get good tips, like where the elevators are in the shopping center!" Elaine has found support through a program for stroke survivors with aphasia. She does not attend a formal support group, but she has met several spouse caregivers through the program, and they have become her friends and emotional supporters. She sees these friends regularly, with and without their stroke-survivor spouses, and sometimes spends hours on the phone with them.

Counseling and Psychotherapy

Emotional support can also come from professionals. Many caregivers have difficult feelings that are hard to handle even when support is available from friends and families. One-on-one professional counseling or psychotherapy for caregivers is very helpful if sadness, anxiety, or other emotional problems persist despite other types of social support, or when difficult feelings are interfering with your daily activities.

Some caregivers hesitate to participate in psychotherapy because they see the need for professional help as a sign of "weakness" or incompetence. Dana Reeve was interviewed about her experience as a spouse caregiver after her husband, actor Christopher Reeve, experienced a severe spinal cord injury. She presented the need for psychotherapy in a different light: "I'm a big believer in therapy. . . . I consider it to be similar to getting a heart doctor for your heart. A therapist is an emotion doctor for your emotions." Emotional or psychological problems are part of the human condition, just as physical illnesses are. And caregivers of stroke survivors can clearly benefit from the support of an "emotion doctor," especially when depression or other emotional problems are present. But counseling and psychotherapy do not need to be the "last resort" or reserved exclusively for times when you are suffering with severe anxiety or depression. Psychotherapy can also be helpful when you simply need to talk to an empathetic, objective person, someone who can give undivided attention to *you* and your concerns. As Rita points out, "caregivers sometimes get overlooked [by medical professionals]. The whole emphasis is on the patient." Jane, another caregiver, notes that her husband's doctors "never ask me how *I* am. It's all about *him*. It's like I'm invisible." Individual counseling or psychotherapy can help when you feel overlooked or overloaded. In addition to providing attention to your concerns in the sessions, psychotherapy can help you learn new behaviors and develop self-confidence to seek the attention you need from doctors and other professionals.

There is a widespread but utterly incorrect belief that all psychotherapy is psychoanalysis, a form of treatment that requires hundreds of hours "lying on the couch." In reality, most therapists working with caregivers today use an active type of short-term therapy that focuses on solving practical problems in the daily life of the caregiver. The therapist helps you find new ways to deal with real-life issues, building your self-esteem and improving your mood.

> Beth had psychotherapy with a social worker she found through a local stroke association. Although she also received support from friends and colleagues, she says that the social worker saved her life. The social worker met with Beth for individual therapy, met with each of the children separately, and held some sessions with the whole family. Beth found this therapy tremendously helpful emotionally, and because her social worker was knowledgeable about stroke, the sessions also provided valuable help with practical problems, such as strategies to improve Wayne's memory and to work out age-appropriate roles for the children in promoting his recovery.

If you seek psychotherapy or counseling, make sure that it is provided by a licensed psychologist, psychiatrist, social worker, or professional counselor. A therapist who has training and experience in working with caregivers or families experiencing chronic illness or disability, and who has some understanding of stroke, will be most helpful. Specialists in rehabilitation psychology and neuropsychology have extensive training in the broad range of cognitive and emotional problems associated with stroke and in the emotional impact of stroke on caregivers. You may be able to find a skilled psychologist or other therapist through your primary-care doctor, your spouse's neurologist or rehabilitation doctor, or other caregivers.

Taking Care of Yourself

Medical Care

Taking care of yourself includes paying attention to your physical health needs and your needs for recreation and relaxation.

Unfortunately, many caregivers tend to ignore their own preventive health care needs. They become so focused on their spouse's health and medical needs that they put their own on the back burner. One of the most important things you can do for yourself is to make time for your own health care. This means getting regular physicals or checkups as recommended by your doctor, mammograms and PAP smears (for women), prostate exams / PSA tests (for men), and any doctor-recommended screenings for eye disease, colon cancer, or other conditions. You might be tempted to put off needed surgeries or medical procedures because you feel pressed for time. But placing yourself at greater risk for illness or disability will not be helpful for your spouse in the long run. When your own health is at issue, consider using respite care or calling in your family or friends to help your spouse while you take care of yourself.

Exercise and Diet

In addition to medical tests and treatments, adopting a lifestyle and habits that promote good health will improve your longevity and the quality of your life and will make you a better spouse and caregiver. Regular exercise lowers your risk for heart disease, diabetes, and stroke; improves your physical strength and endurance; and has the added benefit of reducing stress and enhancing feelings of well-being. Exercise increases your self-esteem by promoting a feeling of mastery over your own body. And exercise stimulates the body to produce endorphins, chemicals that create a feeling of mental well-being, sometimes called the "runner's high."

Making time for exercise means giving yourself permission to focus on your own needs. If guilt (about taking time for yourself) or procrastination is getting in your way, try to remember that even a small amount of exercise can make a big difference in how you feel. Start off with walking or other light exercise for just 10 minutes a day if that's all you can manage. Then gradually add more time as you feel able. Many people like to combine exercise with socializing, for example, walking with a friend or taking an exercise class. The social contact distracts from the "work" of exercise and makes it more fun.

People often skip meals or eat "junk food" when they are stressed. If you have developed this habit, think about how you can change your routine and take time to eat regular meals. Cooking and eating healthy foods is good for your body and can also be relaxing because it forces you to slow down and concentrate on one of life's simple pleasures. Eating a regular dinner with multiple courses (instead of grabbing a "fast food" meal in a paper bag) with your spouse or family also provides a time for socializing, resting, and reflecting on the day. If you have a special diet because of your own medical problems, you may need to experiment with recipes that fit the guidelines your doctor has recommended for you. While this may be different from your spouse's diet, diets lower in sugar, fat, and salt are good for everyone. It is worth taking the time to discuss your dietary needs with a doctor or nutritionist, so that you can prepare and share meals with your spouse that are good for both of you. If you do not like to cook, you can probably find restaurants in your community that are willing to accommodate your own or your spouse's food preferences at a reasonable cost. Eating at a restaurant can be a good way to slow down, have fun, relax, and also get a nutritious meal.

Other lifestyle habits that affect your health include smoking and drinking alcohol. Smoking increases the risk for heart attack, stroke, lung disease, and cancer. If you are tempted to start or resume smoking or to increase the number of cigarettes you are already smoking each day, you may be reacting to anxiety or boredom. Try to find other ways to relax, and work on decreasing the aspects of caregiving—or life in general—that are stressing you. Help is available if you need help to quit smoking. Many smoking cessation programs are offered free or for a nominal charge at local hospitals, community centers, or schools. Some psychologists also work one-on-one with individuals to help them quit smoking.

Alcohol consumed in small amounts is acceptable for most people and may even reduce the risk for certain illnesses; however, too much alcohol is associated with numerous medical conditions, social problems, and cognitive impairment and is especially harmful for people recovering from stroke. If you find that you are reacting to stress by drinking excessively, you should discuss this with your doctor and consider getting help to cut down or quit. Self-help groups (such as Alcoholics Anonymous) are readily available in most communities. As with other support groups, it is a good idea to try out several groups until you find one that is a good fit with your values and needs.

Relaxation and Leisure

Leisure activities and relaxation are major sources of pleasure, and loss of leisure time is a frequent complaint of caregivers and one cause of caregiver burnout. Making time for these activities is one way to give yourself a break from caregiving. Just when you feel you have "no time to relax" is when you are probably most in need of a break! Like exercise, relaxation and leisure can be worked into your routine in smaller or larger increments. If you feel you have only 10 minutes a day, then start with that.

Whether sitting with your feet up, reading a book, meditating, listening to music, or lying down for a catnap, relaxation will help "recharge your batteries" and give your mind a rest. Relaxing your mind completely so that you can take a break from the "chatter" of your own thoughts can be particularly restorative, especially when you are constantly concerned about another person's well-being. Relaxation techniques to help you "turn off your thoughts" can be learned and practiced. Individual therapy, classes, videotapes, and audiotapes or books available in most libraries and bookstores offer information on relaxation techniques such as mental imagery, focused muscle relaxation, and meditation. Even when people practice these techniques for only five or 10 minutes a day, they often feel refreshed and revitalized and experience the "afterglow" of relaxation for a longer period of time.

Of course, relaxation can include any experience that takes your mind off life's stresses and worries: take a bubble bath, read a book, walk the dog, or talk to a good friend on the phone. For many people, relaxation and leisure activities are inseparable—seeing a movie, eating dinner with friends, or getting lost in a crossword or Sudoku puzzle can be relaxing activities.

Some of these relaxation breaks, and others discussed earlier—such as taking care of your medical needs, seeing a friend for emotional support, or arranging respite care for your spouse—require scheduling. Although it may seem paradoxical to have to schedule relaxation time, often it is the best way to ensure it will happen. Here are some scheduling guidelines from *Today's Caregiver Magazine* that may help you plan your own social, relaxation, and leisure times:

- Every *day,* take a half hour to do something you like that is relaxing: practice yoga, meditate, do needlepoint, read.

- Every *week,* spend a couple of hours away from the house at a place you like: a museum, a theater, a mall, a coffeehouse, the library.

- Every *month,* spend an evening out with friends: go to a play or a concert, a movie or a restaurant.

- Every *year,* go on a well-planned (and well-deserved) vacation.

You can tweak this schedule to fit your needs; *any* time you take to relax and unwind will help you keep your spirits up and maintain a positive outlook.

Fatigue and Sleep

Fatigue is a significant problem for spouse caregivers. If your spouse needs care during the night, you may have a hard time getting adequate sleep. Sometimes caregivers are busy at night doing household chores that they can't get to during the day when their spouse requires much of their attention. Caregivers may get stuck in a pattern of being "on call" 24 hours a day when their spouse is in the hospital after a stroke. This pattern of disrupted sleep is hard to reverse once the crisis is over.

Elaine moved into Stan's hospital room while he was in rehab, took over much of his care, and slept on a cot the hospital provided. When she took him home, Stan frequently needed help to go to the bathroom at night, and her sleep was disrupted. Even now, when Stan is able to drive and get out on his own, Elaine finds that she's always busy at night, either helping Stan on the computer or catching up on the mail and bills. "I'm always sleep deprived," she says. "I long for the day when I can come home and have nothing to do."

Sleep deprivation can be a cause of depression, strain, and burnout. Rita is awakened often by Paul's coughing and demands for attention. "Sometimes I feel sorry for myself," she says, "more when I'm tired. I never get a full night's sleep." Many caregivers find themselves in situations like Elaine's and Rita's, staying up too late doing chores, being awakened through the night, or both.

Several possible solutions might help you get adequate rest. If you are not working outside the home, you may be able to adjust your schedule to fit better with the needs of your spouse—for example, napping during the day if you know you will be up frequently at night. If you are working, or don't have a chance to nap during the day because of your spouse's needs, you might hire an aide to care for your spouse several nights a week, allowing you to sleep in another room and get a full night's rest. If, like Elaine, you find yourself helping your spouse with late-night projects, you may need to talk with your spouse and set some limits on your availability. Finally, you can ask a friend or family member to "cover" for you while you take a nap or go to bed early some evenings. Having enough rest will improve your mood, your ability to solve problems, and your overall health. Although you may feel that you are depriving your spouse when you take time "away" from her to sleep, the quality of your time with her will no doubt improve when you are better rested.

While fatigue and lack of sleep can contribute to feeling irritable and sad, the reverse is also true. Clinical depression can cause insomnia (the inability to sleep) or *hypersomnia* (sleeping too much). If you find that you frequently can't sleep even when you've made the time for it, or that you often have trouble getting out of bed in the morning even after sleeping eight or 10 hours, you should discuss it with your doctor. Antidepressant medication often helps insomnia; this medication needs to be monitored by a physician. Sometimes, prescription sleep medications can be effective, as Laura found.

> Laura took Craig home from rehab with a feeding tube and a bladder catheter; he was unable to talk or walk. After months of being a 24/7 caregiver, Laura was unable to relax even when Craig started to improve and she finally had time to sleep. Despite feeling exhausted, she just couldn't fall asleep. Laura started taking a sleep medication prescribed by her doctor, which was enormously helpful. She said, "I had to do that; I needed to rest at some point."

Although prescription sleep medications may help, it is best to avoid over-the-counter sleep remedies unless they are recommended by your doctor.

Caregiver Advocacy

Inclusion in Decision Making

As a caregiver, you are often in the position of advocating for your spouse, whether you are negotiating with insurance companies for coverage, requesting specific therapies or other services from your spouse's medical team, or speaking to other care providers on behalf of your spouse. But caregivers also need to advocate for themselves, or enlist others to be their advocates, so that their own needs and desires are not overlooked. You may need to remind the professionals caring for your spouse that you play a vital role in his care—and that considering your needs will promote better care for him. Sometimes a friend or a relative can act as your advocate, to ensure that your spouse's care plan also takes your needs into account.

> When Craig came home from rehab, Laura was overwhelmed by providing his complex medical care and trying to coordinate multiple medical and therapy appointments. She says, "I was going insane . . . between the cardiologist, urologist, ENT, swallowing tests. Then my sister said 'I'll be your advocate.'" Laura's sister took over scheduling Craig's appointments and negotiating to make sure that his schedule worked with Laura's other commitments and stayed the same each

week. This helped Laura to plan around Craig's therapies and provided regular times she could set aside for herself or take care of other chores.

Laura's experience with caregiving became a "crash course" in advocating for herself, as well. "One of the nurses [from the hospital] called me for feedback and I told her everything I was unhappy with," Laura said. "And things did change. You have to speak up for yourself and your spouse. You have to write down your questions, take notes."

At one point, Laura was concerned because the hospital wanted to discharge Craig prematurely, when she felt that neither of them was ready. She discovered that the hospital employed a Patient Advocate, who could serve as a mediator between families and the hospital staff. She consulted the Patient Advocate, who extended Craig's hospital stay long enough for Laura to get some training in how to care for him at home.

Over time, Laura learned that asking questions and voicing her concerns and ideas was necessary to get the best care for Craig and to make her job easier. For example, by simply asking his outpatient doctor, she discovered that many of Craig's medications could be taken at one time—as opposed to the complex schedule given to her when he first left the hospital. This simple change freed up an hour in her day.

Laura's experience illustrates the importance of speaking up when it comes to simplifying care routines, expressing your concerns or worries about your spouse's medical care, and planning your spouse's discharge from the hospital.

To make sure that your preferences and values as a couple are taken into account, you will also need to express your wishes about the location for your spouse's care. The medical team's recommendations regarding home versus nursing home care for stroke survivors with complex care needs may clash with your priorities and values. Again, you must act as your own advocate.

In general, when a stroke survivor is discharged from an acute hospital or a rehabilitation center, nursing home care is recommended only if he has continuing medical problems, physical impairments, or behavior problems that would make home care unsafe or exceptionally difficult for his wife and family. If you are weighing the option of nursing home care for your spouse, it is wise to consider not only his needs but also what you are able to handle. You might choose temporary nursing home care until your spouse has improved or you can arrange for more help in the home. Or you may prefer to take your spouse home, despite heavy care demands. Living together as a couple may be your top priority, even if it means bearing additional caregiving responsibilities. It is your right as a spouse to care for your partner at home as long as you can provide a safe environment. As we saw in chapter 1, sometimes a caregiver who is eager to provide care at home has to convince the hospital that he has the knowledge, family support, and other resources to do so. And sometimes you need to advocate for yourself—and your relationship—to negotiate successfully.

> Rita Harris was committed to bringing her husband home after rehab, but the rehab team strongly recommended that Paul be transferred to a nursing home, because he needed tube feedings and had severe mobility and cognitive impairments. Rita had cared for Paul years before after a severe heart attack; she knew she could manage, and she had the financial resources to hire an aide. But each time they discussed it, the staff reiterated their recommendation for a nursing home. Finally, Rita came to a meeting with the staff and said, "All right, I've decided to place Paul in the Harris Nursing Home—I've checked it out and it's a lovely place." She laughs, recalling that "it took them awhile to get it—that I was talking about my house!" Finally, the staff gave their blessing to her decision.

Rita's and Laura's experiences demonstrate several important components of advocacy: knowing your rights, using available services, communicating your ideas, and being persistent. By asserting their wishes without becoming hostile, they were able to get more of their needs met. In Rita's case, a sense of humor also smoothed over the negotiations with Paul's medical team.

Understanding Your Rights

Knowing your rights as a caregiver means being familiar with *legal rights,* such as what medical information you are entitled to, what mechanisms you can use to represent your spouse, and what financial benefits you may be eligible for (legal and financial aspects of planning for care are discussed in more detail in chapter 6). Equally important is to know your *emotional rights,* what you have a right to expect for yourself as a caregiver and human being. The Caregiver's Bill of Rights (see sidebar) was developed to validate caregivers' human and emotional needs. Many caregiver programs, manuals, and support groups distribute this document to their members. You may find it helpful to review it when you experience conflict with your spouse, try to reconcile competing demands, or ponder the best way to ask others for help.

Defining Your Role

Another aspect of advocating for yourself is taking charge of how your own role is defined—as a caregiver and as a spouse. Spouses who care for their partners benefit from our society's recognition of the special role of caregiver. Without this recognition, many of the supports and services for caregivers that are now in place would not exist. However, some spouses experience a downside to this social recognition: the assumption—often expressed by medical providers or relatives—that because you are the spouse of a stroke survivor, you will necessarily become the primary caregiver. While nearly every spouse of a stroke survivor provides assistance or care at some point, some spouses object to the caregiver label. You may believe that whatever help you give your spouse after a stroke is simply part of being a good husband or wife. Or you may be in a situation, by choice or necessity, in which someone else is performing a majority of the caregiving tasks, and you are able to concentrate on other aspects of your marital relationship.

Since the balance of spousal and caregiver roles is a delicate one and is different for every couple, you and your spouse have the right to determine how much time and energy you will devote to caregiving and to what extent you will define yourselves as caregiver or care recipient. You have to resist social stereotypes and expectations and instead define your role as a spouse caregiver in the particular way that is meaningful to you. If you want more help with caregiving, you should not allow yourself to be "guilt-tripped" by family members who think it's your duty to do it all on your own. Similarly, you may *choose* to do

A Caregiver's Bill of Rights

I have the right . . .

To take care of myself. This is not an act of selfishness. It will give me the capacity to take better care of my spouse.*

To seek help from others even though my spouse may object. I recognize the limits of my endurance and strength.

To maintain facets of my own life that do not include the person I care for, just as I would if he or she were healthy. I know that I do everything that I reasonably can for this person, and I have the right to do some things just for myself.

To get angry, be depressed and express other difficult feelings occasionally.

To reject any attempt by my spouse (either conscious or unconscious) to manipulate me through guilt, anger or depression.

To receive consideration, affection, forgiveness and acceptance for what I do from my loved one for as long as I offer these qualities in return.

To take pride in what I am accomplishing and to applaud the courage it has sometimes taken to meet the needs of my spouse.

To protect my individuality and my right to make a life for myself that will sustain me in the time when my spouse no longer needs my full-time help.

To expect and demand that as new strides are made in finding resources to aid physically and mentally impaired older persons in our country, similar strides will be made toward aiding and supporting caregivers.

*The word *relative* rather than *spouse* was used throughout in the original document.

it all, and you should be able to feel good about your choice, even if friends or family question your judgment.

Sandy Senor's essay "Tips from a Caregiver Husband" demonstrates that self-definition as a caregiver does not always depend on the amount of caregiving a spouse provides. He describes his extensive and attentive care of his wife after she had a stroke resulting in severe physical disability and the inability to speak; he helped her with dressing, grooming, bathing, personal hygiene, and transportation, as well as doing all the household chores—cooking, cleaning, laundry, and shopping. He says, "Caregiving is a full-time job, 24 hours a day, 365 days a year." He describes getting his training to be a caregiver at the rehab center and getting support from other caregivers via the Internet. And yet, he concludes his essay by saying, "I don't look at myself as a caregiver; I am a husband in love with his wife."

The caregiver role, like many other roles that people play throughout life, is fluid, in terms of both the tasks it involves and its relevance to your self-image. Regardless of how much or how little care you provide for your spouse, you have the right to define yourself as a caregiver on some days and as a husband, a wife, a friend, or a lover on others.

Tapping into Caregiver Resources

Knowing where to look for help and support is critical to giving yourself a break. Many resources for information and support of spouse caregivers are listed in the Resources section of this book. Several national organizations are devoted exclusively to caregivers and their social, emotional, financial, and practical concerns. Help of various kinds can be obtained from them. All of these organizations are on the Internet, and much of the valuable information they provide can be printed from a computer free of charge. If you do not have a computer, you can use one at your public library, where the librarian can assist you in looking up and printing information. Some hospitals and rehabilitation centers also provide computer access to patients and their families.

The many ways to get support for yourself include getting help from extended family and friends, using respite care, attending stroke clubs and support groups, and seeking psychotherapy when needed. Taking care of yourself by attending to your needs for medical care, exercise, nutrition, sleep, relaxation, and leisure will help sustain your health and well-being and give you a break from the demands of caregiving. And advocating for yourself or having others advocate on your behalf can ensure that your rights are respected and your thoughts and needs as a caregiver considered.

If you are taking care of yourself—and allowing others to give you a break—you will have more mental and physical energy to bring to your relationship with your spouse. You will be a better caregiver, avoid burnout, and be more attentive to developing and enjoying your relationship with your spouse. The next chapter redirects your attention to your marriage and how you and your spouse can rebuild your relationship after a stroke.

Practical Tips for Support of the Caregiving Spouse

- Social support is indispensable for success as a spouse caregiver. Ask for support or help from others, and accept offers of help when they come your way.

- Use the sources of support that you are comfortable with; family and friends are available to most people, but support can also come from neighbors, community organizations, stroke clubs, hired aides, and respite programs.

- If you are depressed or need additional help to work out your emotional responses or gain a better perspective on your situation, consider seeking psychotherapy from a professional.

- Take care of your own physical and mental health:

  —Make time for relaxation, exercise, and sleep.

  —Eat a healthy diet.

  —If you smoke, get help to quit.

  —Drink alcohol in moderation or not at all.

  —Schedule time in each day to do something pleasurable for yourself.

- Become an advocate for yourself; practice speaking up to express your opinions and get your needs met.

- Remember that you have the right to define your role in whatever way is right for you.

- Use resources that are readily available for information and support; these are described in this chapter and listed in the Resources section of this book.

CHAPTER 5

In Sickness and in Health

Rebuilding Your Marriage after Stroke

Craig and Laura had been married for 31 years, were both employed full time, and had a grown daughter, when Craig had a severe stroke. Craig had had no medical problems and was unusually active for a man of 58—he was a high scorer in pick-up basketball and traveled extensively for his job. A healthy 53-year old at the time of Craig's stroke, Laura was a librarian, planning to retire soon. Craig and Laura enjoyed dining out, going to the movies, and taking long walks together, and they had an enjoyable sex life. They were often apart because of Craig's travel schedule but liked the balance of time alone and time spent together. In short, they had a close and comfortable marriage.

Craig's stroke started with a "whale of a headache." He went to bed and "must have passed out." Laura thought he would sleep it off, but, she says, "I heard strange sounds coming out of his mouth and realized he was not OK, and I called 911." Craig was taken to a local hospital and then flown to a regional trauma center. He went from the intensive care unit to a regular hospital and then to a rehabilitation unit, where he stayed for weeks. Initially, he had multiple impairments in speech, swallowing, mobility, memory, and vision. He needed a feeding tube in his stomach because he could not swallow and a catheter in his bladder because he could not control his urination. Laura recalls that "it was quite scary. But the neurosurgeon was very positive, and told me what I could expect," that things would improve gradually over time. He gave Laura a sense of hope that carried her through the next weeks and months.

Craig doesn't remember much of what happened before his transfer to the rehabilitation unit. Although he couldn't talk because his muscles used for speech were weak, Craig could understand what people said to him. He could often answer yes or no by squeezing a hand once or twice. When it was time to go home, Craig was still unable to talk, had double vision, used a urinary catheter, and remained dependent on Laura and his nurses for all of his personal care—bathing, dressing, moving in and out of bed and the chair, toileting, tube feeding, and getting his medications. He recalls, "I was mentally ready [to go home] but I needed so much care. The burden fell on Laura because I was basically a wet noodle! All I could do was sit in a chair . . . and I was doing a lot of napping. And medications, oh god—she had to grind up all the medications and put them in with the tube feedings."

Once at home, in addition to handling Craig's complex care, Laura had to arrange to transport him to numerous outpatient therapy and doctors' appointments, and she had to take over managing the family finances, which had been Craig's responsibility before his stroke. She was able to retire a few months earlier than she had planned so she could devote herself to caring for Craig full time.

Like you and your spouse, Craig and Laura found their life suddenly and dramatically disrupted—turned upside down, really. Craig's impairments and the care he required made their situation especially challenging. Yet, the couple was able to adapt and adjust, hang on through the ups and downs of Craig's recovery, preserve what was most valuable in their marriage, and ultimately redefine their roles, activities, and expectations to continue a satisfying relationship.

Build on the Strengths of Your Relationship

The key to [coping with a stroke] is the relationship of the couple going in. If it's good and can be maintained, that's a big part of it.—Mike, husband and caregiver

One of the ways couples coping with stroke can maintain a good relationship is by identifying and building on the strengths of their marriage. These strengths include all the effective strategies that you as a couple have developed for solving your problems, managing your conflicts, reducing stress, communicating feelings, and maintaining physical and emotional intimacy. Probably some of your strategies are practiced by other couples; others are unique to your relationship.

Although it may seem intuitive that building on your strengths will help you cope with a major disruption in your life, it's easier said than done. Sometimes the extreme stress brought on by a stroke brings out the worst in couples—they may find themselves losing their tempers and fighting or arguing more, they may become more distant and uncommunicative with each other, or their mood may be so strongly affected that they aren't able to concentrate or solve problems.

Most couples, if they had a good relationship before the stroke, find that these negative reactions are short-lived, and they gradually return to the constructive coping and problem-solving skills they used in the past. But your relationship may feel so different after your spouse's stroke that it's hard to recall what made things work for you before. You can become stuck in patterns of conflict or distancing and have difficulty reestablishing the feelings of contentment, security, or pleasure that your marriage provided before the stroke.

If you find yourself stuck in this way, try asking yourself how you and your partner solved problems before the stroke. How did you deal successfully with other life challenges? What worked for you in the past? Try thinking about what made your marriage a source of comfort or excitement, fulfillment or fun? What parts of your relationship did you find most valuable and satisfying? Examples might include

- shared activities, projects, or interests,
- the ability to argue and talk things over,
- the ability to fight and make up,
- a fulfilling sex life,
- positive thinking,
- a sense of humor,

- respecting each other's individual needs, and
- cooperating in reaching your common life goals.

You can make a conscious effort to tap into your particular strengths and create opportunities for enhancing the aspects of your relationship that served you well in the past.

The relationship strengths that were helpful to Craig and Laura and to other couples that are discussed in this chapter are intended only as illustrations of what is possible, not as an exhaustive list of relationship strengths. While you and your spouse may have these strengths or may aspire to them, the two of you have, in addition, your own special reservoir of strengths that you can dip into as you start to rebuild your marriage after stroke.

Share the Impact of the Stroke

One of the pitfalls for couples after a stroke is the tendency for each spouse to define his or her individual identity and needs primarily in terms of being a caregiver or a care receiver (discussed in chapter 2). These roles can seem to "take over" your personalities and your relationship, especially when the stroke has a large impact on your daily lives. When the roles become too stereotyped or rigid, your relationship may begin to feel out of balance and unequal, as if your spouse has all the problems and you have to come up with all the "fixes." Your spouse may then feel guilty and sad about being a "burden," and you may feel resentful and burned out. But if you can look at the stroke as something that happened to both of you, and if you can respond to it as a mutual problem, then you may be able to avoid letting your roles as caregiver and care receiver become set in stone.

John Rolland, a psychiatrist and family therapist, notes that when a couple views one partner's illness not as "his" problem, but as "their" problem, it is easier for them to see how the physical and psychosocial impact of the illness affects both spouses. This view empowers couples, as they form a united front and combine their strengths to cope with the illness as a relationship issue. So one of the strengths that can be applied to rebuilding your relationship is the ability to share the impact of the stroke on practical problems and on your feelings.

By working on problems together, you will have more power to solve them.

> Mike and Doris approached their life from the perspective of "we" not "me" and worked together on many projects that other couples might consider either "men's" or "women's" work—putting a roof on their old farmhouse, cooking and household chores, and making financial decisions. When Doris's mother was ill, they took her into their home and shared the caregiving duties. Mike put it this way: "Since we're a couple, we're one and the same. Essentially we're one person."
>
> The attitude of "we" not "me" has served Mike and Doris well in maintaining the exceptionally close relationship they enjoyed before Doris's stroke. They are acutely aware that the stroke affects both of them, and they view recovery as a shared project through which both can benefit. They have applied their combined energies toward this end by joining stroke support groups together and becoming subjects in research projects on stroke at a local university. And they have adjusted their expectations of the future in light of Doris's limitations, pursuing new activities in which they can participate together and finding different ways to "be there for each other."

Dave and Sally supported each other through troubling times even before his stroke. Dave was laid off, after 15 years as a foreman, when his company moved its factory to Mexico. Sally, a stay-at-home mom, "stepped up to the plate," getting a part-time job at a restaurant to help tide them over while Dave searched for employment; eventually, he was hired in another state. When Dave had his stroke three years later, he and Sally rallied the "team spirit" that had gotten them through that earlier difficult period. "The stroke was our common enemy," said Dave. "I was on the front lines, but she was always my rear guard!" They worked together on important decisions regarding work, finances, reassigning roles, and finding new sources of mutual enjoyment.

Be Friends with Your Spouse

Sexual attraction is often the spark that brings couples together and creates the exciting feeling of romance and being in love. This aspect of the relationship is very prominent during courtship and the early years of marriage. But for many couples, friendship becomes as important as sexual love, or even more important, as their relationship develops and matures.

Some spouses begin their relationship as friends, only later developing a sexual attraction and romantic feelings for one another, while others find that the friendship aspect of their relationship grows with time and eventually becomes their primary mode of relating. Still other spouses manage to combine these two aspects of their marriage and others, too, such as parenting, becoming partners in work or business, and sharing hobbies or special interests.

Couples with strong friendship bonds both love and like each other. They can be passionate and romantic but also relate to each other as buddies, or even best friends. They may have an easier time accepting changes in sexuality after stroke, because their relationship is based on friendship as well as romance, and it includes platonic as well as sexual elements. They enjoy hanging out together, talking to each other, sharing experiences, and confiding in each other. They are interested in each other's problems, projects, and ideas.

Rita and Paul were friends for many years before becoming romantically involved. Rita liked the way Paul was "helpful to others, always going the extra mile." She was intrigued by Paul's knowledge of linguistics and history and liked hearing stories about his travels. Since his stroke, Rita's respect and admiration for Paul contribute to the vitality of their relationship, in spite of Paul's many impairments. She likes his sense of humor, his intelligence, and his creativity. Paul likes telling Rita about projects he dreams up—recently, a plan for a research institute and observatory on the coast of France—and Rita is enthralled by these "interesting ideas," even though she knows they will not be realized outside of Paul's imagination.

When you like your spouse, you value her personality traits—including the quirks—admire her talents, and respect her opinions. If you and your spouse enjoyed a close friendship before the stroke, this is an asset for rebuilding your relationship. You may be more comfortable with relying on your spouse for emotional support.

Mike and Doris were close friends and confidants throughout their marriage. Mike can trust Doris to hear him out and respect his feelings.

"She would never put me down if I talk to her about a problem," he says. He values this part of her personality, which he finds "is basically the same" as before the stroke. Mike says he has a tendency to overwhelm himself by starting too many projects at once; Doris was the one who helped him set priorities. Despite her current cognitive limitations, Mike says, "she still keeps me grounded." She helps him stay focused and get things done.

Spouses who like each other and relate as friends tend to admire each other's best qualities and to be more tolerant of mistakes or shortcomings; their friendship can help them maintain a close and positive relationship after a stroke. Toni, for example, describes Luis as "a very smart guy. He's even more observant now [since the stroke], good at analyzing. His intellect is almost 100%." And Mary praises Jim for being a "fighter," whose motivation and inner strength are a constant inspiration for her.

Reframe "Problems" as "Opportunities"

When Eli had a stroke and developed aphasia, he and Janet made a project of reestablishing communication. Eli says, "if there's an obstacle, we get around it." Eli participated in an intensive language program, where recovery became his "full-time job," and Janet became his language "coach." They expect that future problems will stimulate their search for new solutions; Eli notes that "the situation is not static. More recovery is possible."

The ability of couples to solve problems effectively is important to relationship success in general. Effective problem-solving has been linked with better recovery for stroke survivors and a better mood and less stress for caregivers. Often, good problem-solvers are people who look at problems as opportunities for growth and have confidence in their ability to solve them. Couples who view problems in this way may feel more optimistic about their future and believe they will succeed in making positive changes in their relationships. They are less likely to see the stroke as a catastrophe. This confident approach to solving problems was shared by several couples interviewed for this book.

Laura and Craig's "can-do" attitude helped them plan for future needs before Craig's stroke. They tended to face decisions head-on, making choices based on a rational assessment of alternatives, such as opting to enroll in the short-term disability policy offered by Craig's employer. After the stroke, they recognized from past experience that grieving would be inevitable—but they did not believe in "wallowing." Laura recalls that "sometimes he'd be crying and I'd say, 'OK—we're going to give ourselves 10 minutes to cry and feel sorry for ourselves—and then we'll move on.'" They have applied this practical orientation to planning for their "golden" years and the possibility of further disability. Recently they moved into a new house, where the master bedroom, office, and living space are all on the first floor and—although they hope that neither of them will need a wheelchair again—the entrance to the house is fully accessible; if necessary, Laura says, "you could roll right in."

Toni and Luis liked making major life decisions together, usually after enjoyable and stimulating debates. After his stroke, Luis was more inclined to let Toni make these decisions, but she continued to ask him for his opinion; she says, "I want some challenge, I feel he should push back." They continue to share the satisfaction of tackling difficult problems and projects; recently they installed new tiling in their bathroom—by themselves.

Balance Time Together and Time Apart

Another potential strength in your relationship is the ability to keep a good balance between "couple time" and time alone to pursue your individual hobbies, friendships, or relationships with extended family members. If you have few interests of your own or not much of an individual identity outside of your marriage, you may be more frightened by your spouse's stroke and find it harder to cope if he can no longer function in his usual way. If you and your spouse have spent all your time with each other, it may also be more difficult to find support from outside the marriage, because you will have developed fewer friendships and social contacts. Or if you led "parallel lives" and spent little time together as a couple before the stroke, you will find it difficult to cope with the fact that stroke requires, at least initially, a period of intense togetherness and cooperation. Most couples fall somewhere between these two extremes, and the optimal balance between togetherness and separateness for your marriage is not necessarily the same as it is for other couples. Knowing how to recreate this balance is a strength that you can bring to your marriage after a stroke.

Craig and Laura had enjoyed a nice balance of time alone and time together before his stroke. But for some time after the stroke, Craig's multiple impairments made it necessary for him and Laura to spend all of their time together. They soon realized that they needed to have some time apart in order for each of them to feel more satisfied with their marriage. This meant that Craig would need to be more independent for some of his self-care. Laura discovered that she could teach Craig how to do his own tube feedings. She had been setting up the feedings for him, five times a day, and was unable to be away from the house for more than an hour or two. When he learned to feed himself, Craig said, "It freed her up to go out and it gave me a feeling of independence. I started doing it a couple of times a day." In the process, Craig regained some self-confidence and a sense of control over his own body and routine. Laura was able to see her friends or pursue other activities outside the home, and her need for an independent life apart from her relationship with Craig was satisfied.

After the initial period of intense and sometimes frightening dependence that follows a stroke, it is natural for both spouses to have some resistance to increasing independence. Your own and your spouse's fears about her safety, reluctance to lose the heightened sense of closeness that comes with surviving the stroke and its aftermath, or hesitance to reclaim responsibilities put on hold during the initial period of recovery are some of the reasons why couples have ambivalent feelings about greater independence. Not being clear about what your spouse is capable of can also get in the way. In Laura's case, it was when one of Craig's doctors asked if he was doing his own tube feedings that it dawned on her that he might be able to do this for himself. Because she recognized their need for more independence from each other, she took the doctor's comment as her cue to begin fostering Craig's independence in self-care—and doing so allowed each of them to enjoy some time alone.

Josie and Tom liked to "do their own thing" before Tom's stroke, and as soon as Tom could safely be on his own, they resumed this pattern. Josie says, "Some couples are joined at the hip, but we couldn't stand that." While they enjoy going to church and socializing as a couple, they each have their own friends and hobbies. Tom frequently travels without Josie, accompanied by his best friend or one of their sons.

Don't Forget Humor

A sense of humor is invaluable for defusing conflict in relationships, coping with stress, and increasing the experiences of pleasure, fun, and closeness in relationships. If you have relied on humor to get through difficult times in the past, or to create a warm and accepting atmosphere in your relationship, you may find that it is extremely helpful in rebuilding emotional bonds with your spouse after a stroke.

Craig says that after he had surgery to stop the bleeding in his brain, he "accused the surgeon of making me look like a cabbage patch doll; there's a ridge like a newborn has on the top of my head!" Although he now walks without a cane, Craig's balance is poor and his pace is very slow. His speech is intelligible, but when he's tired, he may slur a word here and there. "I walk and talk like a drunken sailor," he jokes. Craig and Laura shared a laugh at themselves as they recalled Craig's progression to independence in the shower and Laura's nervousness about letting him shower alone. Initially, Laura had to come into the shower with Craig and wash him completely. Later, he washed himself sitting in a shower chair; she insisted on staying in the bathroom, but Craig says she kept complaining "about how hot it was in there!" Finally, he was able to take a shower unassisted, standing up, but Laura continued to stand outside the door, unable to relax.

Although Laura has frequently been anxious about leaving Craig alone or letting him try new things, her ability to laugh at her own hang-ups has helped her cope with these anxieties and gradually become more comfortable with Craig's continuing steps toward independence.

Similarly, humor has kept tensions and frustrations under control in Paul and Rita's marriage. Although Paul's memory and other cognitive abilities have been significantly impaired by his stroke, he is often most responsive to Rita when she kids around with him. And she enjoys Paul so much when he exercises his own sense of humor—even after he's been cantankerous or uncooperative. "He'll win me back by being charming or humorous. He still won't do what I want him to do, but he'll try to make me smile." She has learned to see the humor in some of his uncontrollable outbursts, too, noting that he "gives me a hard time but I know he doesn't mean it. Today he yelled at his aide the whole time he was in the shower, like he was being killed, but when it was all over he smiled and said 'Thanks!' He's still funny."

Use Social Supports and Accept Help from Others

Getting support from other people can help couples rebuild their marriage after stroke. Couples who have more social connections are in a better position to get the help they need. But even if your social network is limited, you can probably find a helping hand from within your circle of acquaintances. Family members, friends, and even neighbors often offer their help or are willing to help if asked. Some couples may try to do everything on their own, but this can put extraordinary strain on the caregiver and the relationship (see chapter 4). Getting help can protect your relationship from becoming one-dimensional— all about caregiving and recovery. Assistance with some of the practical aspects of running your household, managing your finances, or providing hands-on care allows you and your spouse to direct more energy toward other aspects of your relationship, such as communication, companionship, and intimacy. You can turn to the same social "assets" that worked in the past: think about who helped you or provided emotional support before the stroke and what kinds of things they can help you with now.

Laura reports that her parents and sister provided periodic respite care for Craig while Laura went to the grocery, did other errands, or gave herself an occasional "treat, like getting my nails done." In the early months of Craig's recovery, her family cooked most of their dinners, allowing Laura to have more time with Craig that was not taken up with doing chores or providing care. Her sister's husband helped Laura learn to manage the bills and finances, and their daughter helped out by organizing Craig's medical history and medication lists, so Laura could have them ready when talking with Craig's doctors.

Change Relationship Patterns That Don't Work

All couples develop a variety of relationship patterns, which are influenced by their personalities, cultural factors, and particular life circumstances. Couples have characteristic ways of dealing with different aspects of their life together—making decisions, doing chores, raising children, romance and sexuality, and coping with illness or other stressors. Most couples find that the relationship patterns in some areas of their married life are smooth and effective, involving closeness and cooperation, and in other areas they are more likely to experience conflict or emotional distance.

Sometimes the pattern of relating in a facet of a couple's life stops working effectively, either because they cannot accomplish their goals (for example, they cannot agree on who should do which chores, so important things are left undone) or because they experience emotional unhappiness in that area (for example, they are unable to feel emotionally close or to share their feelings openly with each other). It may be difficult for couples to confront and change these patterns, especially if they are doing well and feeling satisfied in other areas of their relationship. But a stroke can "shake up" a couple's marriage and highlight areas of difficulty. Patterns of relating that seemed adequate before might not work as well after the stroke. You may have to change patterns to manage the new demands that come with a stroke—to encourage your spouse's recovery, protect your own well-being, and keep your marriage strong despite the losses that come with illness.

Certain relationship patterns, though they might have worked well for a given couple for many years, fail to work in the aftermath of a stroke, and the marriage becomes much less satisfying. For example, your relationship may have been marked by stereotyped or rigid roles and division of labor, emotional distance between you and your spouse, isolation from social connections with family and community, or an imbalance of power, whereby one spouse had much more power than the other over decisions that affected you both.* If the marital relationship patterns that worked for you before your spouse's stroke become problematic afterward, feelings of frustration, unhappiness, or being stuck will probably serve as a signal that something needs to change. You and your spouse can alter some of your relationship patterns on your own, but you may need or may benefit from the assistance of a professional marriage or individual therapist to help you make changes in long-established patterns and achieve the best solutions (see "Getting Professional Help," in this chapter).

Distance and Lack of Communication

In some marriages, spouses share resources, cooperate in raising their children, and attend social events together, but they have little emotional intimacy. Such spouses often enjoy a high degree of independence from each other, while spending much of their emotional energy on close relationships with friends, children, or co-workers. Although one or both spouses may long for more closeness at times, emotional distance may feel acceptable or even desirable when each is busy with work, child-rearing, or other activities that keep them emotionally engaged with other people for many hours a day. If you have had this type of relationship, you may find that after your spouse's stroke, when you are spending more of your days together, the distance between you becomes more noticeable and less tolerable. Some couples find that a stroke presents an opportunity to become emotionally closer, and you may wish to move in that direction. Sometimes a creative approach, with much trial and error, is necessary to establish closeness and connection.

> Before Tom's stroke, he and Josie had a wonderful relationship in most respects. But Josie felt that there was always more distance and less communication than she would have liked. "Tom was in love with his

---

*Some couples have relationships that are dysfunctional or even destructive, because of patterns of emotional or physical abuse, alcoholism or drug addiction, severe mental illness, or other serious problems. If your relationship suffered from problems like these before your spouse's stroke (or if you develop such problems after the stroke), you should consult with a mental health professional; solutions to such problems are beyond the scope of this book.

work," she says. He was often away on business or came home late from the office, and then he wanted some time to unwind—alone. "We weren't like our friends who had happy hour every day after work, to sit down and talk. We never did. He'd come home and read the mail and the paper. I think he felt like, 'I'm tired, why bother?' and I didn't like that." After his stroke, communication was extremely difficult because of his aphasia. They had much more time together after the stroke, but they found that their inability to understand each other was maddening at first. They would often blow up at each other out of sheer frustration, and then there "would be all these days of not talking at all . . . but that doesn't help anything," Josie says. They needed to change a lifelong pattern of distancing from each other when stressed, just at the time when communication was most difficult and stress was unusually high.

Solving this dilemma required spending time together pursuing activities in which their enjoyment was not dependent on conversation. Resuming their physical intimacy, going to concerts and museums, and enjoying family events together helped them feel closer. They were able to travel together, something Josie had always hoped to do when Tom retired. Josie eventually accepted that Tom's speech would not fully recover, and she stopped feeling neglected when he couldn't express his thoughts to her in words. She gradually let go of her hurt and anger, discovering that "peace is very valuable."

Trying to Do It All without Help

As we have emphasized before, one of the strengths couples can rely on in coping with stroke is the ability to get help from others when they need it. But for some couples, a pattern of doing everything with and for each other is strongly engrained. Unlike Josie and Tom, who prided themselves on not being "joined at the hip" but also suffered from a lack of emotional intimacy, some couples build their whole romantic life around the notion of being ruggedly independent and not needing anyone but each other. If you and your spouse have shared such an "us against the world" relationship for many years, then you know that under most circumstances, this pattern meets your needs. But it can put pressure on both of you during times of trouble or stress. After a stroke, this relationship pattern may no longer work, especially if your spouse has multiple care needs. If you have no outside help, your marriage is in danger of being "taken over" by the demands of providing care, leaving you exhausted and your spouse with insufficient social contact and support for recovery.

Alice and Fred fell madly in love at the junior prom and married right after high school. Their parents' strong opposition to the marriage reinforced their romantic notion that they "didn't need anyone, anyway." They moved across the country and cut off communication with their parents. Settling in rural Oregon, miles from their nearest neighbors, they developed a self-sustaining lifestyle; they grew their own food, sewed their own clothes, and made and sold handcrafted wooden signs. After their son was born, Fred got steady work on the early-morning shift at a logging company. He was home by mid-afternoon and spent the rest of his day with Alice. They had little to do with their community and spent all their free time together. Although they took care of their son's basic needs, he often felt shut out by their tight relationship with each other. At age 18, he left for college in the East, married, and settled in Boston. Fred and Alice saw him rarely and had sporadic phone contact. They continued to be intensely proud of their ability to fulfill each other's every need. As soon as Fred was eligible for retirement, he left the logging company and joined Alice in their home-based craft business.

Then at age 58, Alice had a large right-brain stroke. She developed left-side weakness and severe left-neglect (inattention), affecting her ability to read, make crafts, cook, and do many other chores. Sometimes she could not locate her own left hand and it got tangled in her wheelchair. She was impulsive and unaware of safety risks in her environment. Fred had to watch her constantly to prevent her from accidentally injuring herself. She needed help with getting washed and dressed, using the toilet, and even eating, because she ignored the food on the left side of her plate. Fred was soon overwhelmed, and although Alice hated the idea of accepting help from outside their marriage, Fred knew they needed it.

Fred had to "change the rules" in his relationship with Alice in order for their marriage to survive. He swallowed his pride, called their son, and asked for him to help them make a workable plan. Then Fred explained to Alice why a change was needed—that it would be impossible for him to provide her care 24 hours a day and also manage the shopping, cooking, and running of their business and that he was feeling "in over his head" and frightened for her safety. He reassured Alice that he loved her as much as ever and would make sure they always had time together, even though they would need to rely more on other people. By the time their son arrived, Alice was warming to the idea. They were surprised by their son's competence and caring and his willingness to be back in their lives. He helped them make a plan for Alice's care, and he lifted their spirits. Eventually, they moved to Boston to be near him. Fred joined a craft guild, where he made some friends. And Alice had help from her daughter-in-law, a home health aide, and new neighbors. Fred made sure that he and Alice had "only us" time for at least a few hours every day, and on the weekends he stayed home with her, talking, snuggling, relaxing, and recapturing the romance of being "alone together."

Recovery Ups and Downs

Recovery after stroke is an ongoing process, as is the creation and rebuilding of any long-term relationship. Even when things are going well, there are times when life's many ups and downs will trouble you. It is not unusual for a caregiver spouse to have mixed feelings about his marriage—that it feels both gratifying and frustrating at the same time—or to experience waxing and waning marital satisfaction over the course of time. While stroke complications, new health problems, losses of loved ones, and other "downs" of life obviously require emotional adjustments, the "ups" of life are also sources of stress and may necessitate significant new adaptations. Paradoxically, you may experience strong feelings of frustration or dissatisfaction when your spouse shows signs of getting better. Leaps in recovery can upset the balance of your relationship, raise your expectations unrealistically, or create the need to adjust your roles and responsibilities yet again.

Life goes on after stroke, and that means not only a gradual return to prestroke routines and activities but also the likelihood that you will encounter new problems and losses, unrelated to the stroke. One of the "downs" for couples in the process of rebalancing or rebuilding their marriage after stroke is the need to cope with additional crises.

> About two years into Craig's recovery, Laura's mother was diagnosed with advanced breast cancer. Laura's parents needed her help, but she was still afraid to leave Craig alone. The challenge for both of them was to trust in Craig's new physical abilities and to allow Craig to be an emotional caregiver for Laura, after being the care recipient for so long. Craig says, "I tried to give as much as I could. I understood that she wanted to be with her mother every day. And luckily I could take care of myself." This was an emotionally difficult time for Laura, but her need to lean on Craig helped them restore some balance in their marital roles and actually strengthened their relationship.

Changes in Recovery

Among the challenging "ups" that you may experience after your spouse's stroke is the need to cope with changes in your roles and expectations that are brought about by steps toward recovery. Your spouse's increased physical abilities or independence may require additional changes in your and his roles, just as you were getting comfortable with caregiving and care receiving. Improvement in one area of his functioning (such as walking) may raise your expectations for a complete recovery, which can lead to terrible disappointment. Or you might experience a resurgence of grief or sadness about his ongoing limitations in specific areas (for instance, speech and language) that you now see more sharply in contrast with his improvement in other areas.

> Laura says that as Craig has improved—he can drive, walk, talk, eat, and help with many things around the house—she gets "frustrated because I fall back on wanting him to do things that he used to do and that he can't do now. He's gotten so much better, why doesn't he do this?" Craig says that her increased expectations are "almost a sign that she's forgetting my condition," but he recognizes the disappointment this can sometimes create. He has felt frustrated by the contrast between his extensive recovery, on the one hand, and his remaining limitations, on the other. "We're almost back to normal, but there are

certain things I can no longer do and certain things I can do. As you get better, the aggravation factor gets worse—you keep knocking down the targets, but others come up."

Craig and Laura had to learn that this combination of recovery in some areas and ongoing limitation in others is par for the course after stroke. They have come to expect the "aggravation factor" and manage their frustrations by closely communicating with each other about how their situation is changing and how they can best respond to it. They generally keep an open mind about the future—knowing that Craig's recovery may end at any time but staying hopeful that he will continue to improve. And they are ready to "fine-tune" their roles and relationship in response to evolving circumstances and needs.

> Janet and Eli's experience is similar. During the first two years after Eli's stroke, their roles were clear—Janet took over many activities that Eli could not do, and Eli's "job" was to concentrate on his therapies and recovery. Now that he can resume a more equal role in the marriage, they are sometimes surprised and anxious when Eli's impairments "show." Janet sometimes finds herself expecting him to behave or communicate just as he did before his stroke, and then she gets "disappointed at times by his limitations," she says. "I forget that I need to cut him some slack." As Eli's language has improved and he is more often successful at expressing his thoughts and feelings, his failures are all the more exasperating. Janet finds herself worried that Eli's frustration will lead him to "retreat from communication."

Eli's improvement spurred new anxieties about his remaining impairments and a return of Janet's grief and sadness. Although Eli was getting better, Janet's hopes for a return to "normal"—to the way their marriage was before the stroke—became like a mirage of water on the horizon of a desert; each time she thought they were just about to get there, she realized the goal was still far away and perhaps unattainable. She became discouraged and mildly depressed and started working with a psychotherapist, who helped her cope with the situation. In therapy, Janet learned to shift her focus toward the positive aspects of Eli's recovery and to change her thinking about his progress, so she could enjoy his milestones along the road to recovery rather than worrying about whether he was "getting there." These changes in her perspective ultimately helped her get over the hump, and she and Eli have continued to work together on improving his communication and creating a stronger relationship.

Permanent Cognitive Limitations

Permanently damaged memory, verbal communication, reasoning, and judgment may limit the extent to which you can rebuild a marriage based on reciprocity and intimate partnership. Cognitive impairment that decreases your spouse's ability to empathize with you or to comprehend the emotional nuances of speech can also interfere with the process of reestablishing intimacy with your spouse. You may not be able to be as emotionally close to your spouse as you used to be. You may feel despair over the "loss" of your mate, whom you now experience as "a different person." It may feel to you and your spouse as if the prestroke relationship has died, and it is not unusual to experience a sense of grief and loss even as you struggle to create a new type of relationship. Sometimes both partners are held back by all-or-nothing thinking about the marriage—that if it does not return to the way it was before the stroke, then it is worthless. But you may be able to create a different kind of meaningful relationship with your spouse. Here are some things you can do to take care of your marriage when your spouse has significant cognitive limitations:

- Concentrate on sharing activities in which your spouse can participate (and which both of you can enjoy).

- Notice the kinds of emotional and physical connections you can still make with your spouse; think about ways to enhance those connections or create the conditions that foster them.

- Find additional emotional and social support from relationships with friends and family.

- Award yourself credit for what you have accomplished.

- Give yourself permission to redefine your relationship, make new agreements with your spouse, and set new goals.

These strategies may help both you and your spouse to make the most of your marriage, even though it is different from what you had in the past or expected for your future.

Stan's limitations in verbal expression and his reduced capacity for empathy have made it necessary for Elaine to adjust her expectations for their marriage. "I'll tell him my problems," she says, "but he can't really give me feedback. He's a little into himself; he doesn't ask me how I feel." Stan has difficulty delaying gratification and frequently interrupts her. "Whether it's a train of thought or I'm trying to follow a recipe, he'll say 'come on' whenever he needs something. He's just not the person I spent all these years with. He's really different; he's got different issues." Elaine has struggled to accept these limitations, while relishing the better aspects of their relationship. She enjoys the fact that Stan is usually in a good mood and rarely expresses anger or frustration. "He's always upbeat and positive. He's so cute most of the time, it's hard to get mad at him . . . he's always been so easy." Elaine and Stan have found activities they can enjoy together and have regained some of the emotional closeness and sexual intimacy they enjoyed before his stroke. Elaine gets some of the empathy and support she needs from her friends. Her co-workers at her part-time job have provided positive feedback and boosted her confidence and self-esteem. She has also learned to value her own accomplishments more, even when Stan is unable to express appreciation. She reports, "I think I'm beginning to pat myself on my back. I feel a little proud of myself."

Neurobehavioral Problems and Dementia

Neurobehavioral problems after a stroke include a variety of conditions caused by damage to particular areas or nerve pathways in the brain. Included are cognitive, behavioral, and emotional disturbances that result in disordered behavior—that is, behavior that is disorganized, ineffective for completing routine tasks, offensive to others, dangerous, or emotionally distressing for family members and caregivers. Disturbances in *executive function,* or the regulation of behavior, form one set of neurobehavioral problems. Among these problems are

- impulsiveness (acting without thinking about the consequences, sometimes with risks to one's safety);
- a lack of inhibitions (the inability to hold back socially inappropriate behavior, also referred to as *disinhibition*);

- difficulties in initiating (beginning) a particular behavior, in switching between tasks, or in stopping a behavior once it is begun (*perseveration*);

- problems in planning and organizing behavior; and

- difficulty in sequencing (completing tasks in the right order).

Abnormal emotional states can include

- apathy (a generalized loss of interest, concern, emotional experience, and motivation);

- irritability, agitation, or aggression; and

- inappropriate crying or laughing that is not related to the situation or is more extreme than the situation warrants (emotional *lability*).

Severe left-neglect and other types of unawareness of oneself, others, or one's limitations are discussed in the prologue.

Stroke survivors who have primarily one type of cognitive problem associated with stroke, such as memory impairment, aphasia, or visual-perceptual impairment, do not usually have significant behavior disorders. As you have seen in the many examples throughout this book, even people with severe memory loss or aphasia can behave in socially appropriate and effective ways, enjoy a variety of productive activities, and negotiate relationship changes based on mutually understood agreements with their spouses. But when someone has multiple types of cognitive problems, or if they occur in combination with other behavioral conditions, severe disorders in social, emotional, and intellectual function, along with aberrant behavior, can result. Such a combination is the hallmark of vascular (stroke-related) dementia.

Vascular dementia can result from one very large stroke, recurrent strokes involving different brain areas, or multiple tiny strokes that result in cumulative damage to brain function over a long period of time. Vascular dementia is more common in older people. It tends to worsen over time as a result of ongoing vascular disease. In advanced cases it resembles Alzheimer's disease and can result in symptoms of confusion, disorientation, wandering, aggression, or other difficult and potentially dangerous behaviors.

The abnormal emotions and behaviors associated with stroke-related behavioral conditions, including dementia, can be worsened or helped, to some extent, by changes in the environment, life circumstances, or relationships. But in general, these troublesome behaviors are not under voluntary control by the stroke survivor. They are not due to stubbornness or playfulness and do not result from a conscious decision or thought. In addition, the stroke survivor is commonly unaware of having these behavioral problems. This makes them difficult to treat. They do not usually improve with psychotherapy, couples counseling, or negotiation between spouses. It does absolutely no good to blame your spouse if she or he cannot modify these disturbing behaviors, or to blame yourself if you cannot influence or "get through to" your spouse.

However, treatment with medications or behavioral modification techniques may help control some of these behaviors. If your spouse's behavior is disturbing to you or others who interact with him, or if you feel that your spouse's behavior is dangerous to himself, to you, or to others, then it is wise to seek evaluation and treatment by a psychiatrist specializing in neurobehavioral disorders. A psychiatric evaluation can help determine the cause of the behaviors, the best course of treatment, and the most effective strategies for you and your family, or other caregivers, to manage the behaviors at home.

Neurobehavioral problems and vascular dementia create significant barriers to rebuilding a marital relationship. Creativity, patience, and dedication are needed to help keep some parts of your marriage alive. You may be able to experience pleasure or fulfillment in your relationship by redefining your expectations, focusing your attention on the best features of your spouse, and discovering meaning and value in whatever positive interactions are still possible.

Before his stroke, Paul was a talented linguist and teacher. Now he has impairments in memory, reasoning, judgment, and regulating his behavior. He is prone to temper tantrums or fits of anger and to exaggerated expressions of emotion. Rita has taken over all of the organization, planning, financial management, and major decision making for their marriage, as well as initiating much of their communication, social life, and intimacy. She has accepted that their relationship will no longer be fully equal, but she values Paul's contributions to the relationship and stimulates him to use the cognitive skills that he has—

including the ability to tell stories, discuss history, and read. Rita is also able to accept many of Paul's difficult behaviors because she knows he is not able to control them, and she doesn't take it personally. She says, "When he gets angry, he's not mean, just frustrated. Even though he gives me a hard time, I know he doesn't mean it. It's so frustrating for him; he doesn't understand, doesn't know how to help himself." Although he does not always empathize with her stresses or problems, she appreciates his expressions of positive feelings. "He's supportive of me going out by myself, never resentful. He always says 'Have a good time.'" Rita has been able to focus on the best in their relationship, while accepting its limitations. The best times are when "he tells me he loves me, appreciates everything I do, when he's gentle and affectionate." She notes that his cognitive capacities seem to be sharper on some days than others and that "when he's responsive, when he's cognitively there, that really gives me a boost!"

For some couples, however, especially when dementia is advanced, the nature of the marital relationship may be irrevocably altered or even lost. Marital interactions may be limited to providing care for your spouse and to fleeting experiences of connection or shared affection "in the moment." The continuity of the relationship can gradually disappear, so that eventually the person with dementia cannot relate in any meaningful way. In these most severe cases, spouses may wish to continue caring for their mate, but they will need to rely on family and friends to provide companionship, support, and emotional intimacy. The care of a spouse with advanced dementia may be too physically demanding or emotionally wrenching. Or it may be impossible to provide a safe environment at home. In such cases, care in a nursing home can be the best option for your spouse with advanced dementia—and for you. You can continue to help care for her and to maintain a relationship to whatever extent is desirable and possible, while beginning to reshape your own life. Maintaining your relationship with your spouse while she is in a nursing home is discussed further in chapter 6.

Professional Help

Laura and Craig were both depressed in the early stages of his recovery. He "went through two 'why me?' phases—'why did this happen to me' and 'why did I survive?'" Craig also cried easily, and this made Laura feel more depressed because he seemed so upset and she couldn't do anything about it. She was very anxious and was fearful of leaving Craig alone. They went to a psychologist together, and each one also had some time alone with the psychologist. The psychologist helped them "find ways to relax" and helped Laura to trust in Craig's ability to be alone. They were able to improve their coping skills, separately and together, and each gradually recovered from depression.

Sometimes, despite the best efforts and intentions, couples feel blocked in their efforts to get their marriage back on track after a stroke. You may feel as if you're in a rut and unable to move your relationship forward, or you may be caught up in a cycle of arguments or conflicts that you are unable to stop. If you and your spouse are clinically depressed, if you feel trapped in your marriage, if you are relying on alcohol or drugs to "get you through the day," or if there is any physical aggression or emotional abuse in your relationship, then you should seek professional help. A mental health professional can provide immediate relief when you are in a dangerous or threatening situation—for example, by prescribing medication for depression, referring you to an alcohol treatment program, or admitting you or your spouse to a psychiatric hospital if needed (if violence or suicide is a concern).

Marital psychotherapy, perhaps combined with individual therapy, can help you and your spouse to understand and work on changing the underlying causes of the conflicts or unhappiness in your marriage. Some causes might be related to the behavioral problems discussed in the previous section, and you might benefit from learning better behavioral management techniques or trying a different medication for your spouse. If there is emotional or physical abuse, it often stems from unhealthy marital dynamics predating the stroke; the extra stress of stroke and caregiving can push a rocky relationship to a breaking point. Therapy can help you find a way to repair the damage to your relationship and move forward, or possibly to recognize that the marriage is no longer viable.

A licensed psychologist, psychiatrist, social worker, or counselor who has experience with stroke and with couples therapy will be most helpful. You can find a therapist through your physician, your spouse's rehabilitation providers, your state psychological or social work association, or your local community mental health center. If you feel that you or your spouse is in a crisis (having suicidal thoughts, acting erratically, or behaving in a threatening manner), you should seek immediate help at a hospital emergency room or by calling 911.

Of course, it is best to prevent a crisis or impasse from occurring, to seek formal support or counseling before your situation feels intolerable or turns into an emergency. Professional help can be useful at any point when you have difficulty with the process of rebuilding your relationship, or even as a source of ideas to improve on a situation that is already going fairly well. While couples counseling is particularly useful to work on communication and sexuality, individual therapy can also be helpful as you work with your spouse to improve your relationship.

> Tom was clinically depressed after his stroke, and Josie felt she should not discuss her own sadness with Tom because she had to "be up for him." She pretended to feel good even though she was crying often and feeling terrible. She finally went to a therapist, who helped her understand that she was experiencing normal grief and that sharing her feelings with Tom might make him feel less alone. The therapist also emphasized the importance of taking care of herself. She says, "That was the best advice I got from the therapist: if you feel good about yourself, then Tom will feel better. But if you're dragging around and depressed, he won't do well." The therapist told her it was OK to pursue her own activities, rather than "hover" over Tom. She became more comfortable with open expression of her emotions and needs, which led to greater closeness with Tom; at the same time, they gradually resumed the independent activities they had enjoyed before the stroke. Sometime later, when Josie felt "terribly neglected" because of Tom's loss of interest in sex, she again consulted her therapist. "She told me 'You have to seduce him,'" Josie said, "and I thought that was funny." But after thinking about it, she recognized that as before, she was not expressing her true needs or feelings to Tom. When she did express her sexual desire directly, he was responsive. "In time, it worked, things got back to normal."

Find the "Silver Lining"

Every couple, regardless of whether or not they experience a stroke, will inevitably face some physical and emotional losses that come with aging or illness. All couples need, at some point in their lives, to adjust their expectations, give up old roles or take on new ones, and redefine what makes their relationship valuable or satisfying. In the course of normal aging, this process happens gradually. But when one spouse has a stroke, the change is sudden and dramatic, requiring a major readjustment in the marital relationship. Throughout this book, we have described various ways in which you and your spouse can make these adjustments and take better care of your marriage and yourselves. In addition, there are a few characteristics of couples that can help you and your spouse not only to cope adequately, but even to see the "silver lining" in living with a stroke—to interpret your experiences in a more positive way, which in turn will motivate you to continue striving to enhance the quality of your relationship.

Commitment

For many couples, perhaps particularly those who have been married for several decades or more before a stroke, commitment to their marriage vows and to the shared life they have built together is a major reason to continually reinvest energy and creativity in their relationship after a stroke. Whether you feel committed out of love, duty, or a combination of both, if your intention is to stay in the relationship with your spouse forever, you will be more motivated to adapt to the changes in your situation brought about by stroke, to let go of old and outdated expectations and dreams for your relationship and create new dreams, new goals, and new ways to find enjoyment and contentment.

"When you're married, you're married, for better or for worse. A lot of people don't make too much of that today," says Josie. She had been married to Tom for more than 30 years when he had his stroke, and this year they celebrated 57 years of marriage. "Even in the worst of times—during our battles, and we've had battles—how could I walk out?

I couldn't live with myself, because I'm important [to Tom], aren't I? How would he manage?"

In the 27 years since Tom's stroke, they have shared many joyful experiences—the weddings of their children, becoming grandparents many times over and then great-grandparents, traveling to Europe, cruising the Caribbean—and developed new friendships. These shared experiences have strengthened their commitment, even as they continued to cope with Tom's stroke-related impairments. While they stand on the foundations of their prestroke relationship—love, sexual attraction, shared enjoyment of family, immersion in church, and volunteering—they have also added some new layers, which include different ways of communicating, increased emotional intimacy, pride in dealing with adversity together, and a conscious effort to work as much fun as they can into each day.

For Elaine and Stan, married for 50 years, "perseverance, patience, and love" are essential in their ongoing attempts to reinvigorate their marriage since Stan's stroke. Although it has been a struggle, and at times they still feel "very alone," there has never been any doubt about their commitment to each other. Sharing a social life, travel, walking, hobbies, having a sense of humor, and expressing affection have helped them remain "in touch" emotionally. Elaine continues to hope that Stan will recover more of his prestroke abilities: "You can't give up, certainly . . . never say never!" But at the same time, she has accepted that she and Stan have to build their relationship around what is possible now. "You reach a point where you have to be real. Sometimes it takes me a long time . . . but time eases things."

Accentuate the Positive

An effective coping skill for dealing with loss in some aspects of your life is the ability to focus more of your attention on what is not lost, to shine a spotlight on the valuable and enjoyable aspects of your relationship that remain intact. Accentuating the positive side of their experience, while accepting or just not paying as much attention to the negatives, helps many couples view their life after stroke as the glass half (or more than half) full, and not the glass half empty. You can focus on the positive by reevaluating your resources—social, financial, or intellectual—and recognizing that at least in some ways, your situation compares favorably to others'.

> Josie says she feels "so fortunate because Tom had taken out disability insurance before the stroke. Financially we can have these diversions. We've been able to have a lovely lifestyle. We enjoy eating out whenever we want, traveling, living in a lovely community. How many people get to live this way?" Aside from their financial situation, Josie and Tom feel fortunate because his stroke was not as bad as some. "When you look at so many problems people have in this world, like Alzheimer's . . . it can always be worse." Tom agrees with Josie when she notes that their perspective has shifted over time, allowing them to see how far they have come: "It's pretty good—I know that now."

Some couples can appreciate the positive aspects of their relationship after a stroke because they compare their life after stroke to what could have happened—the stroke survivor could have died instead of surviving or could have been left with a more severe disability.

> Laura notes that, "in a positive vein, the stroke brought us closer together. We were a team. He needed me and I needed him. And I was so thankful that he was alive." Craig says, "We were closer because we were so interdependent." Although they have both returned to many of their individual activities, Laura says, "I still feel I have it—I feel closer to him still, since his stroke, than I did before." She also notices a new appreciation for life, "so much more than I ever did [before the stroke]. I appreciate Craig more. I guess you see little things, little changes, and you're so happy and thankful for every little thing you see."

> Wayne, whose stroke resulted in severe and lasting memory impairment, still puts his emphasis on the positive. He notes that he's grown closer to his wife, Beth, as a result of the stroke; he has learned to listen to her and respect her wisdom. "I know that stroke is hard to deal with, but you're alive. You have to remember that you are alive, and try to become stronger." Beth recalls the night of Wayne's stroke, when the doctor told her he might not survive. Even with his current limitations,

Beth sees how far they have come together and values having him as her partner.

Faith and Spirituality

Religious faith or a sense of spirituality is important for many couples. Faith can strengthen a couple's commitment to each other, provide emotional support in difficult times, and serve as a framework for finding meaning in life in general, and particularly in times of adversity. Organized faith-based groups, such as religious congregations, affiliated community centers, or prayer groups frequently offer practical support, such as providing meals, transportation, shopping, or respite care for members who are experiencing a crisis. And they offer a built-in social network, support from fellow members, and guidance from clergy. Whether you practice a religion as part of an organized group or find comfort in individual prayer or spiritual practices, faith may help you focus on what is good, valuable, and meaningful in yourself and in your relationship with your spouse.

Rita and Paul were both deeply involved with their church before Paul's stroke, and they share a strong experience of spirituality. "Faith in a higher power" has strengthened Rita's resolve to make the best of her marriage to Paul. She says, "When I give it over to God I feel more relaxed and confident that I'm doing the best I can." Faith has also helped her find meaning in the struggles she and Paul have faced and to view their situation in perspective, recognizing that others may be even worse off. "In our church they say that if everyone laid their cross on the floor and they were all mixed up and you were asked to go pick one up, you would pick up your own cross to carry. I really believe that you're not given more than you can handle."

Josie and Tom describe themselves as "regular church-goers" and believe that their shared involvement with church groups and services has continued to strengthen their relationship.

Laura found that she experienced greater spirituality after Craig's stroke; "I had more faith in God, I prayed more."

Wayne and Beth found their church community to be an ongoing source of friendship, support, . . . and casseroles!

Hope and Optimism

Along with religious faith, or in its absence, many couples have an attitude of optimism and hope that strengthens their resolve to cope with the effects of stroke on their relationship.

> Rita accepts that her life with Paul will always have its difficulties, but she knows that "there's always light at the end of the tunnel. There are dark days, but then the sun comes out."

Couples can have "faith" in doctors, medical research, supportive families and communities, or their own physical and mental strengths to help the person with a stroke recover more fully. Hope and optimism about the future increases their confidence that life—and their marriage—will continually improve. Cultivating, or tapping into, your reserves of hope and optimism can also help you to see your spouse in a more positive light.

> Toni never questioned whether Luis would recover. "I just thought he should get better. Over the years, he's gotten better and better with his aphasia. Every now and again I forget that he's handicapped." She notes that they both take a consistently optimistic view of their future. "He's so positive. Life's not perfect, but we don't concentrate on the negatives."

Sometimes optimism and hope evolve from an initial positive experience of recovery after stroke or grow from the confidence that couples feel after weathering the early storms of their poststroke relationship.

> Beth notes that right after a spouse's stroke, "you just have no idea what your life is going to be like. I didn't believe it would get better, but it did." Now that Wayne has made significant progress and their relationship continues to be strong and loving, she realizes how important it is "to just stay hopeful, don't lose hope. Because it does change, and it does get better. I remember thinking this is never going to get better. I didn't see it coming because it was so far down the road. This is more than I even dared to hope for." When Wayne was in the hospital the first day after his stroke, "they told me 'don't forget, this is just a temporary situation.' And it was. So that's my one piece of advice—stay hopeful!"

Laura and Craig have come a long way together in the three years since Craig's stroke. Craig has made great strides in recovery. Although his walking remains unsteady, his speech occasionally slurs, and his short-term memory remains impaired, Craig can once again drive a car, eat and swallow, read, and participate in social events. He recently joined a public-speaking club and began playing basketball and running again—"awkwardly, but I can do it," he says. Laura enjoys regular volunteer work, takes art classes, and exercises with her friends. They have a comfortable balance of time alone and time together and are able to provide emotional support for each other. They have resumed their sexual relationship after a long period of abstinence. They chose to move into a community that can provide the accessibility and services they will need as they grow older. Although they continue to struggle with frustrations and anxieties, Laura and Craig take care of their marriage by communicating with each other, having a positive attitude, getting help when they need it, and anticipating the future needs of both of them in planning for their later years.

Looking back on their experience, Laura says, "You have to have hope—I had hope. He's come a long way and I always believed that he would. I believed in Craig." Laura and Craig have been able to share their wisdom with others by volunteering as peer counselors to couples coping with the initial impact of a new stroke. Craig notes, "Now we can tell other couples that today and yesterday were your two worst days. From here on out, it only gets better."

There are many ways to rebuild your marriage after your spouse has a stroke. You can build on past strengths, change patterns that no longer work, manage recovery ups and downs, and cope with permanent limitations. You can seek and find your own "silver lining" after stroke, focusing on how commitment, faith, positive thinking, and optimism and hope can strengthen your marriage and add meaning to your life. If you add patience and persistence to these strategies, you will have the winning combination for rebuilding your marriage after stroke.

Practical Tips for Rebuilding Your Marriage after Stroke

- Try to identify the strengths of your marriage. Think about how you solved problems with your spouse before the stroke and what made your marriage a source of fulfillment and fun. Once you identify these strengths, you can build on them to help you cope with the effects of stroke on your marriage.

- You and your spouse have unique strengths as a couple, but you may also benefit from cultivating some of these strategies, which have helped other couples:

  —sharing the impact of stroke,

  —reframing "problems" as opportunities,

  —balancing time spent together and time apart,

  —having a sense of humor, and

  —getting social support and help from others.

- Think about changing patterns of relating that get in the way of building your relationship. For example, if you have been very distant from your spouse, explore ways to come closer and communicate better. If you have been isolated from others, try to expand your social horizons to include emotional support and practical help from family and friends.

- If your spouse has a permanent cognitive impairment that affects the quality of your relationship, the following strategies may help you maintain a meaningful connection:

  —concentrating on shared activities that both of you can do and enjoy,

  —enhancing the emotional and physical connections you have with your spouse,

  —giving yourself credit for what you have accomplished, and

  —giving yourself permission to redefine your relationship, to set new goals, and to make new agreements.

- If your spouse has severe behavioral problems or dementia, seek evaluation and treatment by a knowledgeable psychologist or psychiatrist. You will also need to adjust your expectations of your spouse and your marriage and try to discover meaning and value in the activities and interactions that remain possible for your spouse.

- When you feel stuck and cannot make progress in rebuilding your relationship, seek professional help. Individual or couples psychotherapy can help you find a way to move forward.

- Look for the "silver lining" that makes your marriage good or even better than before the stroke. Some characteristics that have helped other couples do this are

  —commitment,

  —accentuating the positive in their experiences,

  —religious faith or spirituality, and

  —hope and an optimistic outlook.

CHAPTER 6

'Til Death Do Us Part

Going the Distance with Your Spouse after Stroke

When your spouse has a stroke, your view of the world can change dramatically. Living through the experience of stroke—a sudden, unanticipated, and uncontrollable trauma—shakes up your sense that life is safe and predictable. The experience can lead to feelings of insecurity and anxiety about the future. Even as your spouse recovers and you begin to feel that your life is back on track, you may wonder how you will "go the distance" together, how you can chart a course that will promote better health for you and your spouse, and how to prepare yourself for inevitable changes in health that come with aging.

You may be afraid that your spouse will have another stroke and wonder what, if anything, you can do to prevent it. You may worry about how your spouse will be cared for if you die first—or what will happen if both of you need care. If your spouse needs care in a nursing home, you may wonder how you can continue to be involved in her life—how you will relate as a couple if you are separated because of your spouse's extensive needs for care. You may be afraid that you are going to lose your spouse if his health continues to decline, and you may have questions and concerns about how to handle end-of-life care.

All of these concerns are addressed in this chapter. Learning about how you can contribute to stroke prevention and becoming aware of your options for long-term and end-of-life care will help you feel more confident in your ability to plan for and manage the present and the future as you face issues that all couples confront in the course of a marriage.

Try to Prevent Another Stroke

Having one stroke increases a person's risk of having another. This is because the risk factors that caused the first stroke may still be present—such as high blood pressure, high cholesterol, and diabetes, to name a few of the "heavy hitters." Some strokes are caused by congenital blood vessel or heart defects; once these are repaired, they are not likely to cause any further problems. But most strokes are caused by a combination of factors, including some that cannot be changed and others that can be eliminated, reduced, or better controlled by a combination of good medical care and changes in behavior. If you know how your spouse can reduce her risk of another stroke, you may be better able to support her in adopting healthier behaviors. And if you make these lifestyle and behavior changes for yourself as well, you can reduce your own risk for a stroke or other medical problems, while setting a good example for your spouse.

There are a few risk factors over which you have no control:

- *Age.* The risk of stroke doubles with each decade of life after age 55; 75 percent of strokes occur after age 65.
- *Race.* African Americans have a significantly higher risk of stroke than whites, especially among young adults.
- *Sex.* Men have a higher risk of stroke than women before age 65, but not after.
- *Genetics.* A family history of stroke or heart disease before age 65 in one of your parents makes you much more likely to have a stroke or heart disease yourself.

If you are in one of these higher-risk groups, especially if you have a family history of stroke or heart disease, it is even more important to be aware of the risk factors that you *can* control or change.

Several risk factors for stroke can be completely eliminated from your and your spouse's lives by changing your behavior:

- smoking
- excessive alcohol consumption
- use of illegal drugs, such as cocaine, heroin, or "speed"
- obesity
- physical inactivity (lack of exercise)

Stopping smoking can reduce your risk not only of stroke but also of heart disease, lung cancer, emphysema, and other diseases. Reducing your alcohol use to one or two drinks a day, quitting drug use, losing weight, and increasing your level of physical activity will also help you and your spouse to reduce your risk for stroke as well as for heart disease, diabetes, and many other serious illnesses. In addition, these changes will improve your quality of life—you will have more energy, breathe and move more easily, feel more mentally alert, and experience a heightened sense of well-being.

Making lifestyle changes is difficult for anyone, and it may be harder still after a stroke because of depression (which may decrease a person's interest in changing), cognitive problems (which may reduce one's ability to understand the need to change), or physical limitations that make it more difficult to engage in different, healthier behaviors. But stroke can be a great motivator for your spouse to make whatever changes he can to stay healthy—no one wants a second stroke! You can support your spouse's efforts to change in several ways. To start with, you can be a role model; if you are smoking, drinking too much alcohol, using drugs, overeating, or not exercising, think about making changes yourself. As we mentioned before, staying in good physical and mental shape will help you provide the best care for your spouse after a stroke. Furthermore, if both you and your spouse commit to changing an unhealthy behavior and work on it *together*, your chances of success are greatly improved.

If you find that stopping smoking, drinking, or drug use is too difficult for you or your spouse to do on your own, consider drawing on one of the many self-help and medical programs to help you quit. Smoking cessation programs are available at many local hospitals, and 12-step groups such as Alcoholics Anonymous and Narcotics

Anonymous hold free meetings throughout the country. Your insurance may cover treatment for alcohol or substance abuse in an outpatient or inpatient program, if this is necessary.

Information on dieting and exercise is available from many sources, but a stroke survivor should consult her doctor before beginning a diet or exercise program, to make sure the program is safe and appropriate for her specific medical problems and needs. While exercise is beneficial for most people, your spouse may have a medical condition that makes some types of exercise unsafe. A personalized exercise program, designed by a physical or occupational therapist, will help your spouse increase his strength and flexibility and improve mobility and self-care skills, in addition to helping to prevent another stroke. Ask your physician for a referral.

When you are trying hard to change old patterns of behavior, especially if you enjoyed them (even though they were unhealthy), you can improve your chance of success by replacing them with other activities or behaviors. You might spend more time socializing, sample restaurants that serve "heart-healthy" meals, adopt new hobbies or crafts, or enjoy more time outdoors, to name a few. If you are trying not to eat fatty or sugary foods, make sure you have plenty of healthy food and snacks in your house, and experiment with new fruits and vegetables to keep your meals interesting. Trying new recipes and planning healthy meals with your spouse is another way to take the emphasis off "dieting" and increase your pleasure in taking care of yourselves.

Some medical risk factors for stroke probably can't be eliminated, but you can control them to some extent through diet, exercise, proper use of medications, and regular medical care:

- diabetes
- high cholesterol
- high blood pressure (hypertension)
- heart disease (including atrial fibrillation, heart valve disease, coronary artery disease, congestive heart failure, and others)
- clogged or narrow arteries (atherosclerosis)

If your spouse has any of these conditions, she should be carefully monitored by a doctor. Diabetes, high cholesterol, high blood pressure, and many heart conditions are best controlled by a combination of medications *and* the behavioral changes discussed in previous paragraphs. Some heart conditions may also be treatable with surgery or other procedures.

You can help your partner by making sure you understand his medical conditions, are familiar with his medications and how they are to be taken, and have clear and specific recommendations from his medical care provider regarding his diet and exercise requirements and restrictions. Your spouse's doctor (or his nurse practitioner or physician's assistant) should be able to answer your questions about your spouse's stroke risk factors, medical conditions, and treatment regimens and advise you on how to reduce the risk that he will have another stroke. For general guidelines, the American Heart Association's dietary recommendations and stroke prevention tips are helpful; more specific information on reducing risk factors can be found in the book *Life after Stroke: The Guide to Recovering Your Health and Preventing Another Stroke* (see the Resources section of this book).

You can play an important part by encouraging your spouse to take her medication as prescribed and to stick with her doctor's recommendations for dietary changes and exercise. As we said in chapter 1, communication and emotional closeness in families are linked to better compliance with medical recommendations. So if you communicate clearly with your spouse about why you want her to take her medications, and if you regularly express your affection and concerns for her health, you are likely to have a positive impact on her behavior. Remember to praise your spouse when she follows the recommendations to eat right and exercise. Being praised for the right behavior helps a person change bad habits much more than being criticized for the wrong behavior. If the stroke survivor has a poor memory or other cognitive problems, you may need to play a larger role in organizing and administering her medications, planning her meals, and scheduling times for her to exercise. Taking responsibility in these arenas is well worth the effort.

The comedian George Burns once said, "If I knew I was going to live this long, I would have taken better care of myself!" Because modern medicine has done so much to extend people's lives—*despite* the abundance of unhealthy behaviors in our culture—it is tempting to think that if you just take your medicine, you can live to a ripe old age. And while taking pills will help your spouse live longer, his *quality* of life (and yours) will be vastly improved by making changes in health behaviors.

Maintain Your Overall Health

You can also take steps to improve and maintain general good health for both you and your spouse. First, as we emphasized in chapter 4, make time for your *own* health care, in addition to caring for your spouse. Have regular physical exams, including preventive measures such as vaccinations and screenings for cancer, high blood pressure, and diabetes. Follow your medication or other treatment regimens. Make changes in diet and exercise that your doctor recommends. Keep yourself well!

Do the same for your spouse: he should continue to have regular checkups with a family doctor or internist and follow up with his neurologist or other doctors for issues specifically related to his stroke. You can help reduce his disability and promote optimal health for him by paying attention to new symptoms and seeking treatment for medical conditions that may be unrelated to the stroke (such as arthritis, asthma, cancer, and allergies) or mental health conditions (such as depression or dementia). A person who has had a stroke is more vulnerable to the harmful effects of infection, so you must closely follow your physician's recommendations for pneumonia vaccinations and annual influenza vaccinations.

To improve and maintain physical and mental health and well-being, both of you can also

- stay socially active (visit your friends and grandchildren, go to a senior center, attend religious services, join a book or garden club);
- keep your minds active with mentally stimulating hobbies (reading, doing crossword puzzles, making crafts, woodworking, making home repairs, cooking);
- do some physical activity every day (join a formal fitness or physical therapy program, take walks, clean house, garden, ride a bicycle);

- include some time for humor, jokes, and laughter in every day, and keep a sense of humor about your own situation; and

- express your affection to each other (say "I love you," kiss, hug, cuddle).

Whether you are concerned with physical strength, mental acuity, or sexual intimacy, the old adage "Use it or lose it" applies. If you and your spouse make a conscious effort to stay active both physically and mentally, you will give yourselves a marvelous gift: the finest chance of living longer, remaining lively and energetic, and enjoying good health and physical function. And if you include humor, affection, and the social support of friends and loved ones in your life, you can more easily manage stress, experience less anxiety, and enjoy the pleasures of life.

Plan for Your Future Health Needs

In my opinion couples should make plans ahead of time just to be safe, because you never know. Luckily, we had done all the financial planning—long-term-care insurance, short-term disability, long-term disability.—Craig, stroke survivor

Of course, no matter how hard you try to reduce your medical risk factors and improve your odds of a healthy future, there are forces over which you have no control. For most people, there comes a time when declining health, impairment of memory or cognitive abilities, or severe physical disability result in an increase in dependency, with a need for care and assistance from others and perhaps a change in living situation. You and your spouse are likely to experience more medical problems as you age, and even if you are young and healthy, you might have concerns about who will take care of your spouse if you become ill or incapacitated. Planning ahead for your potential needs can greatly reduce your uncertainty and worry about the future. Craig, for example, had signed up for the full menu of insurance options offered by his employer, so there was no interruption in his income when he had his stroke and could no longer work.

Not all employers offer as many options as Craig's employer did, but it is helpful to know what kinds of financial benefits are possible. Some of them may be available at an extra charge through your employer, your union, or some other organization, or you may be able to purchase them individually. There are several areas in which a little advanced planning can go a long way toward increasing your sense of security and control over your future. Here are some questions you may be asking yourself, and some answers in the following paragraphs: *Who will take care of my spouse if I become ill or disabled? And who will be my caregiver?*

Your preferences for care, the availability of an alternate caregiver in your immediate or extended family, and your finances will make a big difference in answering these questions. If your spouse is unable to manage without your daily care, you must (in discussion with your spouse if she is able to participate) designate another person who can assume her care in case you become incapacitated, or you must make other advance arrangements for her care, taking into account her and your preferences and resources. It may be possible to prearrange admission to a particular nursing facility or group care home for your spouse, in the event that you become ill and temporarily unable to care for her.

You might also want to make advance plans to have you and your spouse cared for *together,* in case you develop a health condition that requires care. There are two parts of this scenario to consider. One involves planning ahead for the assistance that you and your spouse may need in the future—who will care for you, where you will receive care, and what kinds of services will be available for you. The other is designating a person who can act in your stead to make medical and financial decisions for both you and your spouse if you are temporarily or permanently unable to do so.

In planning for your ongoing care, there are several options to consider. For some couples, getting care from their adult children, whether in the children's home or in their own, is desirable; many families have a tradition of providing care to older relatives and do not see this as a burden. Living with your adult children can have many social benefits and can be economically advantageous, allowing multiple generations of a family to pool their resources. However, this arrangement will probably work more smoothly if you discuss with your children in advance the specific plans for how you will share expenses, whether you will have a guest room or a "mother-in-law apartment" in your child's home, how your transportation needs will be met, and so forth.

Another option is moving into one of the growing number of life care communities, which provide multiple levels of care in one building or campus, including independent-living apartments, assisted-living services, and nursing home care. Such communities often offer on-site medical care and have amenities such as group dining, entertainment, fitness rooms, transportation services, and community outings. Residents may initially move into an independent apartment but are assured of getting assisted-living services (help with medication management, bathing, and dressing) or nursing home care if and when they need it, in the same building or campus.

> When Josie and Tom reached their 70s, long after Tom's stroke, Josie began to wonder what would happen to them if she got sick. Her children are not likely to provide "hands-on care," and "Tom's not going to be waiting on me hand and foot," she said. "He [would rather] pay someone to do the chores." They moved to a life care community, where, if Josie becomes ill, there will be plenty of help available. They can get meals, laundry, housekeeping services, and assisted-living services if needed; there is an on-site nursing home also. And they like the fact that there are built-in opportunities for socializing and entertainment.

Life care communities provide a great deal of security, but they are expensive and not everyone can afford them. A similar but less costly option is a senior housing complex that includes an assisted-living component (you and your spouse could both get assistance with dressing, bathing, medications, and meals) but does not offer on-site nursing home care. Another possibility is to remain in your current house or apartment and hire someone to assist you and your spouse, either full time or part time. You might use hired caregivers for some tasks and rely on your children or other family members for others. Finally, you may decide to opt for nursing home care for your spouse if you become physically unable to provide his care at home, and to make other arrangements for your own care, depending on the extent of your needs.

Soon after Rita married Paul, he got a new job and they moved far away from the town where they both had grown up. Paul soon had a heart attack and later a stroke; Rita has been his caregiver for many years. Now that she is in her 70s and has developed some medical problems of her own, Rita wonders how long she can keep it up. "Can I really handle this? It's expensive having an aide. What choices will I make when I can't help him?" Realistically, Rita knows that Paul "would need a nursing facility." She says, "I've looked into a facility back in our hometown, because his brothers are there." Rita plans to move with Paul, so she can visit him and live near her old friends.

While she has yet to make arrangements for her own care, Rita will probably find it easier to make those arrangements in their old hometown, where she has some friends and in-laws and some familiarity with local service agencies. Ultimately, moving into the nursing facility with Paul may be an option. Federal law requires that nursing home facilities allow married couples to share the same room, if one is available.

Nursing home care is expensive, and some couples who have the financial means prefer to spend their money on in-home care or assisted living. Medicare does not cover long-term nursing home care, although it will pay for a period of nursing home care if it immediately follows a hospital stay. After that, the care must be paid for out of your personal income, assets, or long-term-care insurance. Once your financial resources are exhausted, nursing home care is covered by Medicaid/Medical Assistance. If you are paying privately for nursing home care and eventually use up your funds (a process called "spending down"), Medicaid will begin making payments to the facility. This means that your spouse can continue to stay in the same nursing home indefinitely; but you may be left with very limited resources for yourself, should you need nursing home care in the future.

Medicaid pays a relatively low rate for nursing home care, so if a person has to rely on Medicaid from the start of her nursing home stay, her options regarding choice of facility and location within the facility may be limited. However, if your financial resources are very limited from the start, nursing home care may be the only affordable option that provides the level of services your spouse needs. To find out more about how to apply for Medicaid and determine your best options in planning for nursing home care from a financial standpoint, consult an elder-care lawyer or seek information from an advocacy group such as the Family Caregiver Alliance or the Alzheimer's Association (see the Resources section of this book).

Health Care Proxy

You need to think carefully about whom you want to trust with the substantial responsibility of acting on your behalf if you are not able to make medical decisions for your spouse or yourself because of dementia or for any other reason. If a person in this situation has not designated a particular individual, then health care providers or hospitals will typically ask his "next of kin" (usually his adult children) to make these decisions for him. If you do not have children, if your children are still minors, or if you prefer not to have your children make medical decisions for you and your spouse, then you will need to identify another person. Obviously, that person should be someone you trust, who understands your values and wishes and is willing to act on your behalf. She or he should know your feelings regarding end-of-life care, emergency resuscitation, and other sensitive medical issues. The health care agent's duty is to make the same decisions regarding your (and your spouse's) health care that you would make if you were able. That person should honor your wishes even if those actions conflict with his or her own desires and beliefs. Creating a written record of your wishes, such as a living will, can help your health care agent understand your specific desires regarding your own medical care and more faithfully adhere to them (see the section "Planning for End-of-Life Care" in this chapter).

Once you have decided whom to designate, you will need to complete a legal document, called a Health Care Proxy or Health Care Power of Attorney, which gives that person the legal right to act as your agent. When your health care agent presents this document to a hospital or a doctor's office, she or he will have the right to get information about your medical care and to make medical decisions for you, *if* you are not able to do so yourself.

Health Care Proxy forms are readily available from any legal office and on the Internet. These are legal documents. What they are called and how they are organized vary slightly from state to state; you will need to use the correct form for your state. It is advisable to complete this form even if your next of kin will act as your health care agent. You can, for example, act as your spouse's health care agent, and one (or more) of your children can be listed as "alternate agents" in the event that you are not available. You can designate a particular child (or children) to be your health care agent and one (or more) other child, a sibling, or a parent to be your alternate agent or agents. Your health care agent can be a friend, if you choose, rather than a family member. Your agent can act on your behalf (or as an alternate on behalf of your spouse) only if you are unable to make your own decisions. As soon as you recover, you again become the decision maker for yourself and your spouse.

Insurance

Can I get financial help to pay for my spouse's care? Can we afford long-term care? How will I take care of myself if we spend all our savings on my spouse's care? Who will manage our finances if I can't do it anymore? How much financial support you have to provide care for your spouse or yourself depends on several factors—your income and savings, what type of medical insurance you have, and whether you have disability or long-term-care insurance policies.

Medical Insurance

Most people under age 65 are insured by private insurance plans, usually purchased through their employer, which cover a portion of their medical expenses. The amount of expenses and types of services covered vary tremendously among insurance plans. Some people are covered by Medicaid, or Medical Assistance, which is a government insurance program for low-income families that is run by the individual states. People over 65, or younger people who are permanently disabled and receive federal disability benefits, are usually covered by Medicare, a federal government insurance plan; most people on Medicare obtain a private supplemental or Medigap insurance policy, which covers some of the costs not paid by Medicare. Medicare subscribers who have very low incomes can get their supplemental insurance through Medical Assistance.

You may have become very familiar with the specifics of your spouse's insurance plan after his stroke, when you had to find out whether rehabilitation, in-home care, or other services were covered. If your spouse has recently had a stroke, his medical or rehabilitation social worker or case manager can help you understand the benefits of his insurance and disability plans. In planning for the future, you will want to find out what benefits your spouse can anticipate after age 65 and to read the fine print on your own insurance policy. If you need assistance in deciphering the sometimes complicated language of your insurance policy, you can call the customer-service number on your insurance card or your employer's human resources office and ask to have someone walk you through the policy and answer your questions. Your spouse will probably be limited to the coverage his current policy provides; it is difficult to switch plans after having a stroke. But if you are healthy, you may be able to switch now to a different plan (such as one that provides more rehabilitation or personal aide services), so that you will have more benefits if you become ill or disabled in the future. You should not cancel your current plan until you have investigated the coverage and the costs of the new plan and have confirmed that you will be accepted by the new plan. Seek the advice of an attorney if you have unanswered questions about insurance coverage or benefits.

Disability Insurance

Disability insurance plans are designed to provide income to a person who is no longer able to work because of a disability. How the income is used is up to you; you may need it for general expenses, or you may be able to use some of it to pay for your long-term-care needs. Social Security Disability Income (SSDI) is a government program that provides income to people who become disabled before age 65. To be eligible, you must have worked for at least three years and contributed to Social Security. The amount you receive is based on how much you contributed to Social Security during your working years.

Private disability insurance is also offered as an employee benefit by many large employers. While you can buy disability insurance as an individual, you are likely to get a substantial discount if you buy a policy through a union or a professional or consumer organization.

Even if your spouse does not have this insurance, you may want to consider buying it for yourself, to help provide a steady income should you become disabled in the future. Disability insurance usually provides a percentage of your income, for as long as you are disabled, until you reach age 65. At that point, Social Security retirement income replaces disability payments. Purchasing disability insurance while you are young is generally a good investment, compared to the risk of losing everything if you have a serious illness. If you become disabled temporarily because of an accident or surgery, short-term disability insurance can provide income while you are out of work.

Long-Term-Care Insurance

Long-term-care insurance policies can provide coverage for nursing home care, assisted-living care, and home-based care. The cost of this insurance depends on the level of care you choose; the greater the coverage you choose (for example, retaining the option to select nursing home, assisted-living, or home-based care), the larger the premium. If your spouse has this type of insurance, she may be able to receive insurance payments toward the cost of nursing home care without having to use up her savings (to become eligible for Medicaid / Medical Assistance). You may wish to consider applying for long-term-care insurance for yourself, if you anticipate that you will need more funds to cover your own care in the future.

Having your own disability and long-term-care insurance allows you to count on some financial help if you need long-term care, regardless of your spouse's situation or how much of your shared savings you may have used. The combination of medical insurance, social security, other disability payments, savings, and pension income allows most middle-class families to make ends meet and obtain adequate care, even when both spouses need care at the same time. For couples who have very limited financial resources, or who have depleted their resources by paying for care privately, nursing home care can ultimately be covered by Medicaid. Under the Medicaid Waiver Program, funds may be available for care at home by a personal attendant (aide) as an alternative to nursing home care; this program requires a special application, and there is typically a long waiting list.

Because there is so much complexity and variability in insurance plans, and because each couple's financial situation is different, you may benefit from professional consultation as you plan for your and your spouse's future care. A Certified Financial Planner or an elder-care lawyer can assist you in analyzing your finances and help you come up with the best financial strategy to maximize your chances of affording the care you need in future years. There are many books that can help you better understand the financial aspects of long-term care, and organizations such as AARP, the Administration on Aging, and the Centers for Medicaid and Medicare Services (CMS) can help you sort out some of the complexities (see the Resources section of this book).

Power of Attorney

You may also be concerned about how your money will be managed if you become unable to make or to carry out financial decisions. Especially if your spouse is unable to participate in managing your finances, you need to designate someone to manage your money on your behalf. This could be the same person you designate as your health care agent, or a different person. You can select more than one person to act as power of attorney, and you can designate an alternate.

There are two significant aspects of designating a person to act in your stead in financial matters. The first one is simple: filling out a legal document called a Durable Power of Attorney, which gives the individual the legal right to manage your finances if you are not able to do so (there are various types of power of attorney; some place restrictions on the scope of financial decisions and transactions the person can perform). The second is more complicated and important: having a series of discussions with the person selected as your power of attorney about what kind of care you want if you become incapacitated, where you want to be cared for (at home, at a relative's home, or at a nursing facility), whether you are concerned about saving money or not, how you feel about selling your home, and other financial decisions.

Elaine and Stan moved to an accessible apartment, close to walkways and parking, so they can remain independent even if one of them becomes more disabled. But Elaine says, "I'm afraid if something happened to me, who would take care of him?" Stan was not able to get long-term-care insurance, but they have a retirement fund. Elaine told her daughter, "If something would happen to me, my wishes are that we could take some of the retirement money and get Stan an aide, so he could stay in the apartment. He likes it here and he doesn't like 'senior' places."

Elaine's instructions to her daughter are very clear regarding her and Stan's preference for him to be cared for in his own apartment, if at all possible. But like many caregiver spouses, her plans for her *own* care are less clear. Even though it is difficult to focus on the care that you want for yourself, you need to think about it. The more detail you can provide to your children or whoever else will be responsible for carrying out your wishes—for yourself and your spouse—the better.

Many people find that their children are afraid of having this discussion. It is hard for your children to think about your becoming ill, especially when you are the caregiver for their other parent. You will almost certainly have to take the initiative in discussing the matter; including a third party (such as a Certified Financial Planner, a lawyer, or even a close family friend) may make it easier for your children to accept the necessity of making care arrangements and may keep the discussion from becoming too emotional.

While it is not necessary to share all of your financial information with your child (or other person whom you appoint as power of attorney), it is very helpful if you can provide him or her with information about where your bank and investment accounts are located, where you keep your checkbook, and so forth, so that she or he can easily step in if you have an emergency. If your spouse managed all your finances before his stroke, you may have experienced the frustration of trying to take over this job without having the right information at your fingertips. This happened to Laura, when she discovered that Craig had done all the banking on his computer, "and all the passwords were in his head." Luckily, Laura had help from the couple's bank and from her brother-in-law in managing their financial affairs. Laura advises other women to "know about your finances," and she says that now they keep all these details written down in a safe place—so if she needs assistance, it will be easier for her daughter to step in than it was for her.

You may be more comfortable having a list of your accounts on file with your attorney or your Certified Financial Planner or in a safe-deposit box. If so, be sure that your power of attorney knows whom to call or what bank to go to so he or she can find the information when it is needed and will be able to get access to your list of accounts.

Power of Attorney and Health Care Proxy forms should be kept on file with your attorney, in case you or your agent misplaces your copies. But both you and your designated agent(s) should have copies at home in a readily accessible location. If you are hospitalized for any reason, you should take along a copy of your Health Care Proxy to be put in your hospital chart, so that your providers will have no doubt about whom to consult if you are unable to speak for yourself. If your spouse is not your health care agent, you can still request that she be given updates about your condition, if you wish.

Nursing Home Life

How do I maintain my marriage when my spouse is in a nursing home? Can I continue to play an active role in my spouse's life? The extent of your spouse's (and your) disability and care needs will play a major role in where and how you receive care. Although many people prefer to be cared for in their own home for as long as possible, that may be impossible, even if funds for home care are available. A nursing home can be the best place for someone with stroke-related dementia, very severe physical disability after one or more strokes (such as paralysis of both arms and legs), or a stroke-related neuropsychiatric condition that results in unsafe behavior (see discussion in chapter 5). But even if you have identified a good facility and determined how you will pay for his care, having to put your spouse in a nursing home can be emotionally wrenching. It is difficult to live in separate places and not sleep together at night. And it may be hard to give up your role as your spouse's primary caregiver and turn over the bulk of responsibility for his care to strangers.

Maintaining a Relationship When Your Spouse Is in a Nursing Home

The type of relationship you have with your spouse when she is living in a nursing home depends on factors such as your spouse's cognitive abilities, your ability to visit, and how much time and energy you wish to focus on your marriage. Some spouses spend many hours a day with their husband or wife in the nursing home, virtually living there during the day and going home only to sleep. Others spend much of their day at jobs or other activities and visit their spouse in the evening or on weekends.

Because of severe impairment, your spouse may no longer recognize you or communicate in any meaningful way. In that case, you may want to continue visiting often just to be with him, perhaps holding his hand or singing or reading to him. Or you may feel that you and she get little benefit from these visits, and you may choose to visit less often and instead spend more energy beginning to build your own life. If your spouse is declining cognitively, there may be a gradual transition between the time when you make every effort to enhance your relationship with her and the time when you step back a bit, refocusing your energy. Even then, in the later stages of their husband's or wife's dementia, many spouses wish to maintain whatever connection they can and to provide the kind of loving care and comfort for their spouse that no one else can.

Making a Home away from Home

When your spouse moves into a nursing home on a long-term basis, one of the toughest things to get used to is the institutional "feel" of the place, which includes standard décor and set times for meals, medications, baths, and bedtimes. One way to help your spouse adjust to living in the nursing home, and to enhance your enjoyment of the time you spend there, is to personalize his room as much as possible. You can bring photographs of you and him (and other family members), favorite blankets and pillows, knickknacks, and other personal items. You can also bring food from home and share some meals together at times you choose, rather than following the nursing home's schedule each day. Usually, the staff will be happy to allow you to provide some of your spouse's personal care, as long as you can do so safely. Even if the staff is providing the bulk of your spouse's care, you may want to develop a routine of personal care tasks that enhance your feeling of intimacy with your spouse: you might shave him, comb or braid her hair, help with exercises, or help your spouse change into pajamas and get ready for bed at night. Personalizing your spouse's room and establishing your own daily routine as a couple will help make the nursing home feel more like your own place and set the stage for more positive interactions.

Staying Close Emotionally

Your emotional connection to your spouse will be enhanced by regular expressions of affection, talking, and enjoying meals and other pleasurable experiences together. It is helpful to find some privacy for yourselves. If your spouse has a private room, this will be easier. If not, you can ask the staff to help you find a quiet area, away from other residents, where you can visit with each other. If you are able to take your spouse outside in nice weather, visiting in a garden or courtyard area or taking a walk in the neighborhood can be a way to get some private time. If your spouse is able to leave the facility and you are able to transport him without help, you may be able to go together to a restaurant, a park, or some other place where you can share some time and enjoy an activity together. If your spouse is able to participate in complex or abstract discussions, you can inform him about current family issues, decisions, or problems and seek his input. If he is not able to process these types of discussions, you can still tell him about events in the family, about your daily activities, or about what is happening in your neighborhood. You may want to read to your spouse, show him pictures or videos of family events, listen to music together, or reminisce about good times you shared in the past.

Expressing physical affection is another way to stay close with your spouse. Touch is not only pleasurable but can be calming for people who are confused or upset. Kissing, hugging, cuddling, and holding hands with your spouse help you maintain your special intimate connection as a couple.

Sexual Intimacy

Maintaining a sexual relationship with your spouse who is in a nursing home can be challenging. Most nursing home residents share a room and thus have little privacy. And many nursing home staff members are uncomfortable with the idea of residents' having an active sexual life. There are several potential reasons a well-meaning staff member may feel this way, and you can better interact with her if you have some understanding of her concerns. Some people believe (incorrectly) that older or disabled people are or should be asexual; they may consider sexual activity in disabled stroke survivors to be strange or inappropriate. Others may feel embarrassed about being asked to help get a person ready for sexual activity (for instance, by transferring the person to bed in the middle of the day or providing additional bladder care). Still others may be concerned that you would be exploiting your disabled spouse by having sexual relations with her or that sexual activity could be physically or emotionally harmful. As we discussed in chapter 3, these are misconceptions and should not dissuade you from experiencing physical intimacy with your spouse. Staff members who have these views are misinformed about aging, disability, and sex.

Indeed, federal laws require that nursing home residents be granted the same rights they would have as private citizens in their own home, including the right to conjugal visits (unless a doctor says this would be medically dangerous). Recently, more nursing home administrators have actively supported residents' right to privacy and sexual expression. If you want to have sexual relations with your spouse in the nursing home—or just to enjoy the physical intimacy of being in bed together and cuddling or kissing without onlookers—you can request access to a private room. Or if your spouse has a private room, you can request that his door be kept shut and that you not be disturbed for a specified period of time. Discussing this with the staff ahead of time, soon after your spouse is admitted, is a good idea. You may want to ask the staff which times of day are most convenient for them to provide privacy. Such communication will give them an opportunity to prepare ahead of time for what you have requested and will show your respect for the professionalism of the staff.

Plan for End-of-Life Care

One of the most difficult things for couples to do is to plan for their care at the end of life and to acknowledge that death will inevitably come. Although many couples believe they know which of them will die first, the truth is that no one can be sure of this. Your spouse may be much older than you, he may have had multiple strokes, or he may be in the end stage of a terminal illness, and yet you may die unexpectedly while he is still alive. How long any one of us will live is one of life's greatest mysteries.

You and your spouse can prepare for the end of life in a couple of ways. One is to make sure that no matter which one dies first, the other one will be left with adequate financial support. The other is to make decisions about the kind of care each of you wants to have at the end of your life. If your spouse is not able to make these decisions, you will have to do your best to make them for her.

Life Insurance

Life insurance policies are one way to make sure that each of you will have a financial cushion if the other dies first. Many people do not purchase life insurance because it can be expensive and does not benefit them personally. In many families, only the primary wage earner buys life insurance, on the assumption that his spouse is dependent on his income and will need it after his death. But life insurance is available to people regardless of their employment history; the cost of the insurance is usually based on the person's age and health history.

As a caregiver spouse, having a life insurance policy on yourself is one way to provide funds for your spouse's continued care if you should die before him; your life insurance money might make it possible for him to be cared for without depleting his other assets. If the stroke survivor did not have life insurance before her stroke, she may not be able to get it—but it is worth exploring the possibility with an insurance agent or through a group such as AARP. If your spouse dies before you do, her life insurance policy will supplement your income and contribute to the cost of care that you need in the future.

Wills

A will (or last will and testament) is a legal document that specifies how you want your money and possessions to be distributed after you die. In your will you can specify that your assets be used to care for your spouse or for any other specific purposes. If you have few assets (for example, you do not own a house and have only a savings account and an Individual Retirement Account [IRA]), you may be able to draw up your will using forms you obtain on the Internet or through a legal-aid service. But it is best, if possible, to get advice from an attorney to be sure that your will accurately reflects your wishes and that it can stand up to any challenges in court. There are also tax issues and estate issues that an attorney or Certified Financial Planner can assist you with.

Ideally, both spouses should create their wills before either one becomes terminally or critically ill. In that way they can avoid having to deal with this practical matter when they are physically and emotionally stressed and might not be able to make important decisions. However, if your stroke-survivor spouse does not have a will but has the cognitive ability to make one, you should consider getting this done as soon as possible. If he dies without a will, settling his estate will be more difficult, and more of his assets may go toward paying fees or taxes. In addition, when you are in the midst of grieving, having to struggle with complicated financial issues can be overwhelming.

In a similar way, it is best to plan for the kind of care you want at the end of life while you and your spouse are still relatively healthy. When you are caught in a crisis, it is hard to think clearly, and you may tend to make decisions impulsively or out of desperation. When you are well, you can make sounder and more rational decisions about the care you want.

Living Wills

A living will (sometimes called an advance directive) is a legal document that spells out the kind of care you wish to have if you are terminally ill and not expected to recover, and if you are too ill to speak for yourself (for instance, if you are unconscious or too confused to make crucial decisions). In a living will, you can specify whether you want to receive life-sustaining treatment if your death is imminent. Life-sustaining treatment includes, for example, receiving water and food through a tube, having a breathing tube put in your throat for mechanical breathing, and cardiac resuscitation. The best way to ensure that your wishes are met is to make a living will and *also* explain your choices to your personal physician and to your health care agent. If your spouse has a living will, be sure to bring a copy of it with you each time she is hospitalized and have it handy for health care providers who may come to your home.

Some hospitals have advance directive forms available, which can be filled out by patients upon admission to the hospital—but patients are often too ill to make those decisions by the time they go to the hospital, so we strongly advise you to complete the forms while you are well. They can be simple and general or quite detailed. Some forms ask for additional end-of-life care preferences, such as whether you would like music played in your room, whether you request visits of clergy or hospital chaplains, and so forth. You may be able to specify the wording of your living will, but in some states the wording is fixed by state law, and you can only select from set options on the form.

When you and your spouse make your living wills together, you have a unique, albeit unsettling, opportunity to discuss your values and wishes regarding end-of-life care. You can work out your disagreements and address your fears about the end of life. Once the living will is completed, you will have a better understanding of each other's wishes and increased confidence in your ability to carry them out.

Hospitals and health care facilities probably will not have ready access to a copy of living will or Health Care Proxy forms that you gave them in the past. Even if the hospital does have copies of the forms from a previous admission, the hospital cannot and should not assume that there have been no changes in your wishes in the meantime. To be sure that these documents are included in your current medical record, you have to bring them with you *each time* you are admitted to a hospital or nursing home, even if you have been a patient there before.

Do Not Resuscitate Orders

A Do Not Resuscitate (DNR) order is a document your doctor signs stating that if you have a cardiac or respiratory arrest (your heart stops beating or you stop breathing), you do not want to be resuscitated or kept on life-support machines. The specifics may vary, and you may be able to choose to have some life-sustaining interventions but not all. Some people want to be resuscitated and given the chance to live as long as possible under any conditions, even if doctors consider their case hopeless. But many others prefer to "let nature take its course"; they refuse resuscitation when death is imminent and when resuscitation would result in prolonged suffering, a poor quality of life, or the possibility of remaining in a coma with no hope of recovering.

If your spouse is no longer able to make medical decisions, his doctor will consult with you about DNR orders. If your spouse has written a living will or discussed his wishes with you previously, it will be much easier to decide what to do. Even then, however, end-of-life care decisions can be wrenching and filled with conflict and uncertainty. It may be helpful to make these decisions with input from other loved ones, trusted friends, clergy, and medical providers.

Hospice Care

Hospice is a program of care for people who are terminally ill (when a doctor estimates that they will live no more than six months), for whom medical care cannot bring about a cure, and who no longer wish to have medical interventions to extend their lives. Hospice provides comfort care to patients, such as pain medications, and provides emotional support to families. Hospice care is often associated with cancer patients, but hospice can help anyone who is near the end of life because of disease or injury.

Hospice care is offered in hospitals, freestanding residential care facilities, or at home. If you have been the primary caregiver for your spouse, you may be able to continue caring for her at home. The hospice nurses will visit periodically, oversee her medical care, and assist you in making final arrangements. Although choosing hospice for yourself or your spouse is a frightening prospect, hospice care is experienced by most families as compassionate, comforting, and supportive.

Anticipating the Loss of Your Spouse

When your spouse becomes terminally ill, you begin the difficult process of anticipating his death and, to some extent, preparing for the new stage of your own life that will follow. While this process is an emotional one for everyone, it may be even harder if you have spent months or years of your life as his primary caregiver. When you leave the nursing home, hospital, or hospice, exhausted after a long day of sitting at your spouse's side, you may feel relieved. But you may also feel a profound sense of loss as you return to an empty house with no one to look after. It is natural to anticipate the grief you will feel when your spouse is gone. And while all spouses wonder how they will relate to the world after they are widowed, you face the additional question of how to define yourself when your life no longer revolves around caregiving.

To make this final stage of your marriage more meaningful for you and your spouse, consider doing some of the following. If your spouse is able to communicate with you, try to stay emotionally involved with her as much as possible. Try to have time alone with your spouse. Think about the experiences you have shared, and talk with her about what you value and cherish about your marriage. This is the time to resolve old hurts and disagreements, to forgive each other for past mistakes, and to let go of any bitterness you have over missed opportunities. It may feel awkward trying to say goodbye to your spouse; instead, you might think about what you would want to say to your spouse if this was your last chance to talk to her—and make sure you say it. You may be able to say it again, or think of more things you want to say, if you have more time together. If your spouse is not able to communicate with you, it will be helpful to talk with another family member or close friend about your relationship with your spouse and your feelings about the impending loss.

You might begin planning for what will happen when your spouse dies. This can be a series of discussions you have with your spouse or with other family members. If you have not made funeral arrangements, now is a good time to do so. Although it is very hard to plan a funeral for your spouse ahead of time, it is even harder to do so immediately after his death, when you are likely to be emotionally overwhelmed and exhausted. Talking about funeral arrangements together, the two of you, gives your spouse the opportunity to express his wishes and may help him and the rest of the family to face the inevitable.

Making plans to have support for the period immediately after your spouse's death can be helpful, for example deciding that you will stay with your son or your sister, or that a friend will stay with you for a week or two. Having such plans in place can relieve some of your anxiety about how you will cope.

Finally, this is a good time to take stock of your work as a caregiver and remind yourself of all that you have accomplished. If you tend to be critical of your performance or feel guilty that you have not done enough, remember that there are no perfect caregivers and try to have compassion for yourself. You have done your best, and you deserve credit for the love and care that you've provided. Your spouse undoubtedly had a better life after his stroke because of your efforts. You may want to make a final assessment of your spouse's needs, to see if there is anything else you can—or want to—do for her. And as death approaches, you may need to let go of being a caregiver, to let others take care of you and your spouse as you share this last stage of your marriage.

Practical Tips for Going the Distance

- *Try to prevent another stroke.* Be aware of and minimize your spouse's (and your own) risk factors for stroke. Take medications as prescribed to control high blood pressure, diabetes, and other conditions. Follow your doctor's recommendations for diet and exercise. Quit smoking, don't use "street" drugs, and consume alcohol in moderation or not at all.

- *Maintain your health.* Get regular checkups, medical screenings, and preventive care, including pneumonia and flu vaccines, as recommended by your personal physician. Keep physically and mentally active. Stay involved with friends and community. Express your affection verbally and physically. Exercise your sense of humor and include some time for fun in your schedule every day.

- *Make plans for long-term-care needs.* Consider buying disability, long-term-care, and life insurance. Use the government benefits that you and your spouse are eligible for: Social Security Disability, Medicare, or Medical Assistance. Consider consulting an elder-care attorney or a Certified Financial Planner to make the best use of your financial resources for long-term care.

- *Make plans for someone to care for you (and your spouse) if you become ill or disabled.* Think about where you want your spouse and yourself to get care; consider a life care community, an assisted-living center, in-home care, moving in with a family member, or nursing home care. Choose trusted persons to act as your health care agent and power of attorney. Discuss your wishes and plans for care openly with those individuals and make sure you are confident that they understand and will honor your wishes.

- *If your spouse is in a nursing home,* maintain your relationship by visiting, sharing enjoyable activities, going on outings, expressing affection, and communicating about important decisions or events. Participate in your spouse's care as much or as little as you like. You have the right to request privacy for intimate time together and to continue your sexual relationship.

- *Make plans for end-of-life care.* Writing your living will and your will while you are relatively healthy and your mental abilities are intact will make it easier for your doctors and loved ones to carry out your wishes. If you or your spouse become terminally ill or have a condition that severely limits quality of life, talk to your doctor about a Do Not Resuscitate order and whether to consider hospice care.

- *When your spouse is near death,* allow yourself to anticipate grieving. Make plans for the funeral. Think about what you will do when he is gone. Make sure you have support from family and friends. Try to wrap up "unfinished business" with your spouse if you have the opportunity—focus on reviewing what you have shared and let go of old hurts or angers. Give yourself credit for all you've done to take care of your spouse and your marriage, and try to accept that there may be nothing left to do. Allow your loved ones to take care of you; you will need them more than ever during this trying time.

From This Day On

The Future of Caregiving

Unlike adult children or siblings who care for a loved one after a stroke, a spouse has a unique connection to the stroke survivor, including the expectation of reciprocity, shared resources, and sexual intimacy. Caregiving on some level has always been woven into your life with your spouse; and yet, after a stroke, for your marriage to thrive, you need to set limits on caregiving and define yourself as more than a caregiver to your spouse. At the same time, it is helpful not to lose sight of the fact that you are now a caregiver with a capital C, with duties and responsibilities that go beyond the normal expectations of a wife or a husband. Recognizing yourself as this special kind of caregiver is an essential step toward finding the education, guidance, and support you need to successfully manage your dual roles.

Fortunately, caregivers are increasingly recognized by our society as a group with special needs, and the resources available to meet these needs are expanding rapidly, as we will see in this chapter. It is equally important for *caregivers* to recognize the significance of their role not only in society at large but also in their relationship with their spouse, their family, and their wider circle of extended family and friends. Acknowledging your own value as a caregiver allows you to take pride in the job of caring for your spouse. As with any job you do, you will perform better if you reward yourself for your accomplishments, celebrate major milestones, and accept help from others when you need a break.

Your family and friends who are not primary caregivers can—and should—recognize and support you in your efforts to care for your spouse. Because more people today have had personal experience with a family member who needs care, there is an increased awareness in many extended families of both the value and the difficulty of being a primary caregiver. Families and friends are often willing to pitch in by sharing some of the regular caregiving tasks, providing respite for the caregiver, helping with unanticipated problems or emergencies, and offering emotional support.

Caregivers Then and Now

Throughout the ages, people have cared for their seriously ill or disabled spouses. But most people born a century ago (your parents or grandparents) did not use the term *caregiver* to describe the role they played in caring for their ill spouses; caregiving was viewed as simply an extension of their role as a husband or a wife. The perspective has changed dramatically in recent years, and *family caregiver* is a commonplace term in families, medical care programs, politics, literature, and throughout all sectors of society.

This change has come about for several reasons. For one thing, improved medical and rehabilitative care has made it possible for people to survive and live for many years after sustaining injuries that in the past century would have been fatal, or with chronic diseases and disabilities that would previously have resulted in a dramatically shortened life span. Stroke care is a good example—up until the middle of the 20th century, little was known about how to treat or prevent stroke, and rehabilitation after stroke was in its infancy. But today the picture is very different. Advances in stroke diagnosis (such as CT and MRI scans) and new medical treatments for stroke (such as tPA, discussed in the prologue) have led, for many people, to improved survival, increased recovery, and less severe disability following a stroke. Advances in stroke rehabilitation techniques reduce medical complications after strokes and improve function and quality of life for many people who have had strokes. Because of these medical advances, there are now more spouses providing care to a stroke survivor, and probably over a longer period of time, than in previous generations.

A second factor in the emergence of caregivers as a recognized social group is the development of rehabilitation techniques, including those that family members can be trained to use, and advances in home care equipment. Spouses can now play a more dynamic and central role in the recovery of their loved one after a stroke. Unlike spouses in earlier times who may have been limited to "hand-holding" and custodial care, today's spouse caregivers are actively involved in physical, cognitive, and psychosocial rehabilitation of their mates after stroke. This expansion of the caregiver role has been influenced in recent years by additional factors: shorter hospital stays after stroke, earlier discharge to outpatient rehabilitation programs, and restrictions in insurance coverage for some rehabilitation therapies. These developments have led many spouses to assume their caregiving role earlier in the recovery process, when the person who had a stroke needs more complex or time-consuming care.

Although not all spouses are comfortable with the caregiver label, recognition of the caregiver role and of caregivers as a distinct social group has been beneficial to today's caregivers in many ways. Caregivers are recognized as a group that makes a valuable contribution to society, both economically and socially. As such, they are also recognized as a group with special needs and rights of their own. One outgrowth of this social recognition is the burgeoning of self-help groups for family caregivers and the inclusion of caregivers in stroke clubs and support groups for stroke survivors. At the same time, there has been an incredible expansion of the information available to caregivers through books, magazines, and the Internet. In addition to providing information on every aspect of stroke and stroke caregiving, the Internet is another source of social support, via numerous chat rooms, bulletin boards, and personal stories shared by caregivers.

Finally, not only are there glimmerings of change in health insurance to support more in-home care services for people with stroke and other disabilities, but also caregiver needs are increasingly considered by health care reformers and social and public health policymakers. In short, caregivers have come out of the shadows and are clearly recognized as a social entity. With this recognition has come an expansion of education, information, support services, and interventions for caregivers, aimed at making their jobs easier and improving the quality of their lives. Caregivers are also helping themselves and each other, through self-help groups and political advocacy. They are a more visible group and, increasingly, a more empowered group.

What's Being Done to Help Caregivers?

Support groups

Caregiver support groups have become widely available throughout the United States. Many hospital-based family and spouse caregiver groups address general issues of caregiving across disease groups. And there are also many support groups designed specifically for caregivers of stroke survivors, young stroke survivors, or stroke survivors with aphasia. You can find such groups through your local chapter of the National Stroke Association or the American Stroke Association, or through a hospital or rehabilitation facility that treats people with stroke. Most of these groups are led or facilitated by a professional social worker or counselor.

Psychotherapy

As the population of people with disabilities—and their caregivers—has increased, more mental health professionals have specialized in understanding and addressing psychological and social problems that affect caregivers. It has become easier for spouse caregivers to find a psychotherapist who recognizes the unique problems of caregivers and has the expertise to treat them effectively. Some psychotherapists use structured, time-limited therapies specifically designed to address the psychosocial problems associated with a medical condition. These therapies can be used in individual therapy with the caregiver or the care recipient or in couples therapy. Psychotherapy that focuses on improving active problem-solving skills and promoting the use of social supports is helpful for many caregivers. And psychotherapy using cognitive-behavioral methods is particularly effective for treating depression. Psychologists with special training in rehabilitation or neuropsychology provide therapies that combine help in coping with the emotional aspects of being a caregiver and help with managing specific cognitive and behavioral impairments that affect your spouse and your relationship after stroke.

Psychosocial Intervention Programs

Many researchers are working to develop new evidence-based programs of intervention for caregivers. "Evidence-based" means that the programs are proven to improve caregiver health, mental health, or quality of life or to promote better outcomes for care recipients. Unlike psychotherapy, these programs are designed for groups of caregivers and are potentially more cost-effective. They are structured—which means that they include specified amounts and types of treatments—so they can be duplicated in multiple geographic or practice locations. As these programs pass muster in research trials around the country, more of them will become available to the general population of caregivers.

The most effective caregiver intervention programs are those that

- address *multiple* stressors and problems affecting caregivers;
- are *flexible,* that is, can be adapted to meet the specific needs of individual participants;
- include a *psychological* or *counseling* component (in addition to education and support); and
- provide a *therapeutic dose* of the intervention (enough intensity, frequency, and/or duration to be effective).

One such program is the New York University (NYU) Caregiver Intervention, for caregivers of people with dementia. It was designed to improve caregivers' coping abilities and to delay (or prevent the need for) institutionalization of the spouse who has dementia by improving support and reducing family conflict. The intervention includes individual and family counseling sessions, weekly support groups, and telephone counseling on an as-needed basis. This program has effectively achieved its original goals and has reduced depression in participating caregivers.

Other caregiver interventions are part and parcel of new approaches to delivering medical care, which recognize the role of family caregivers in the health care team and strive to provide better patient care by educating and supporting caregivers. One of these interventions, currently under study at Johns Hopkins University, offers a program for family caregivers led by specially trained nurses and includes individual assessment of caregiver needs; education and referral to community resources; individualized coaching and assistance with caregiving problems; a six-week self-management class that teaches caregivers how to be better problem-solvers, take better care of themselves, and communicate more effectively with the health care team; and an ongoing support group. This caregiver "package" is embedded in a larger program of coordinated, comprehensive medical care for the care recipients, called Guided Care. Guided Care strives to improve the quality of care and to reduce medical complications for care recipients with multiple medical problems.

Other such programs being developed and tested around the country include Caregiving for You, Caregiving for Me, which is an education and support program, and the Coping with Caregiving class, which focuses on caregivers of people with cognitive impairments. You can find out more about caregiver intervention programs through the Family Caregiver Alliance or the Rosalynn Carter Institute for Caregiving (see the Resources section of this book) and from major university research centers on aging, rehabilitation, and public health.

Researchers are examining caregiver interventions to see how their effectiveness can be improved. They are considering, in addition to the four essential ingredients listed above, the *timing* of interventions, the differences in response to interventions by caregivers from various *ethnic groups,* the varying needs of caregivers depending on their *relationship* to the recipient (spouse, adult child, and so forth), and the *diagnosis* (or behavioral characteristics) of the care recipient. More evidence-based intervention programs designed specifically for spouse caregivers of stroke survivors will surely become available in the near future. A promising development for stroke caregivers is the design of intervention programs intended for delivery over the telephone, reducing the need for travel to a central location to participate in counseling and support sessions. These programs are helpful to caregivers who have difficulty in getting away from home and cost less than face-to-face intervention programs. They include problem-solving and supportive interventions for stroke caregivers and have produced some promising results. Problem-solving and coping programs for caregivers are also being designed for delivery over the Internet or by videoconferencing. Similar programs will likely come to be offered by more community hospitals and rehabilitation centers.

Finally, as new research demonstrates that many caregivers experience psychological *benefits* associated with caregiving (such as a greater appreciation of life or increased self-esteem), interventions are likely to focus on promoting the positive consequences of caregiving, in addition to preventing the negative ones.

How Are Spouse Caregivers Helping Themselves and Each Other?

Some spouse caregivers, in addition to attending a support group, or after "graduating" from one, feel that they have developed some expertise in caregiving or in coping that they would like to pass on to others. Sharing your wisdom with couples or caregivers newly affected by stroke can be very helpful for them and also beneficial for you. If, like several of the couples interviewed for this book, you want to become involved in volunteer peer counseling, opportunities can be found through your local National Stroke Association chapter or stroke rehabilitation hospital.

Spouse caregivers or couples dealing with stroke can also serve as speakers for local stroke groups; you and your spouse may have a particular contribution to make, such as how you coped with aphasia, dealt with depression, or managed a complex insurance issue. Caregivers contribute articles to various stroke-related magazines and other magazines devoted to health or aging. Reading these articles can give you a variety of perspectives on caregiving; writing them can allow you to share your own views and experience and help other caregivers. You can also reach out to your peers or learn how your peers are coping through Internet blogs or social networking sites. (A blog is an Internet journal, where you can write about your own experiences and share them with others on your own Web site.) Some caregivers post articles they or others have written about caregiving, offer caregiving tips, and provide links to resources they have found particularly useful. A social networking site, such as Facebook or MySpace, is an Internet club that allows you to make connections with other members to share photographs, videos, articles and commentary, announcements, computer links, and other information. Increasingly, organizations as well as individuals are members of these sites.

What Does the Future Hold for Spouse Caregivers?

As the spouse of a stroke survivor today, you probably have more complex caregiving tasks to perform, and you will continue to be a caregiver longer, than spouse caregivers of previous generations. While that might sound like bad news, it's also good news, because it means your spouse survived his stroke—and he can be expected to live longer and experience a more extensive recovery and fuller participation in society than was conceivable a generation ago. It is likely that your spouse will improve—somewhat or a great deal—over time, and you will be able to have a meaningful relationship with her, in which caregiving is only one part of the picture.

There is much to be hopeful about. Stroke researchers are working actively to develop new treatments, rehabilitation techniques, and prevention strategies. Doctors who care for patients after a stroke are more aware of how much caregivers influence medical and rehabilitation outcomes, and the role of spouse caregivers as vital partners in stroke care is increasingly acknowledged by the spectrum of stroke care providers. There has been a surge of interest in the psychosocial aspects of caregiving; researchers and clinicians from medical, psychological, and public health backgrounds are working together to develop new methods to promote and support caregiver health and well-being. The mental health needs of caregivers have attracted the attention of psychologists on a national level; in 2009, the American Psychological Association convened the Presidential Task Force on Caregivers, which sponsored the Presidential Symposium on Caregivers at its 2010 national convention.

Many disability and caregiver advocacy organizations are lobbying for changes in our health care delivery system that would create more financial support for in-home care and more help for family caregivers in the form of training, respite care, and social support. This movement is likely to gain momentum as the ranks of caregivers grow and the baby boomers become senior citizens.

Caregivers of the future will certainly not be alone, nor will they be doing their work quietly behind the scenes. Caregivers will become an ever larger, better organized, and more recognizable group; their central role in promoting the recovery of their spouses will be unquestioned, and their political clout will grow. Caregivers, in short, will become increasingly empowered with the tools and support they need to do their jobs—taking care of their loved ones and themselves and nurturing their most important relationships.

Notes

Prologue

p. 19, "About 29 million": Family Caregiver Alliance, "Selected Caregiver Statistics Factsheet," www.caregiver.org.

Introduction

p. 25, "uplifts": Jennifer M. Kinney and Mary Ann Parris Stephens, "Hassles and Uplifts of Giving Care to a Family Member with Dementia," *Psychology and Aging* 4, no. 4 (December 1989): 402–8.

p. 25, The phases of stroke recovery: Jill I. Cameron and Monique A. M. Gignac, "Timing It Right: A Conceptual Framework for Addressing the Support Needs of Family Caregivers to Stroke Survivors from the Hospital to Home," *Patient Education and Counseling* 70 (2008): 305–14.

p. 33, The beneficial effect of caregiving: Stephanie L. Brown, Dylan M. Smith, Richard Schulz, Mohammed U. Kabeto, et al., "Caregiving Behavior Is Associated with Decreased Mortality Risk," *Psychological Science* 20, no. 4 (2009): 488–94.

p. 36, Emotional strain as a risk for older caregivers: Richard Schulz and Scott R. Beach, "Caregiving as a Risk Factor for Mortality: The Caregiver Health Effects Study," *Journal of the American Medical Association* 282, no. 23 (December 1999): 2215–19.

Chapter 1. The Secret Ingredient

p. 42, Social support as a predictor of stroke outcomes: Gert Kwakkel, Robert C. Wagenaar, Boudewijn J. Kollen, and Gustaaf J. Lankhorst, "Predicting Disability in Stroke: A Critical Review of the Literature," *Age and Aging* 25 (1996): 479–89.

p. 45, Brain-swelling evidence from mice: Kate Karelina, Greg J. Norman, Ning Zhang, John S. Morris, Haiyan Peng, and A. Courtney DeVries, "Social Isolation Alters Neuroinflammatory Response to Stroke," *Proceedings of the National Academy of Science USA* 106, no. 14 (2009): 5895–5900.

Chapter 3. A Fine Romance

p. 77, Importance of psychological factors in sexual function after stroke: Juha T. Korpelainen, Pentti Nieminen, and Vilho V. Myllylä, "Sexual Functioning among Stroke Patients and Their Spouses," *Stroke* 30 (1999): 715–19.

Chapter 4. Give Me a Break

p. 93, Interview study on spouse caregivers: Ursula E. Coombs, "Spousal Caregiving for Stroke Survivors," *Journal of Neuroscience Nursing* 39, no. 2 (April 2007): 112–19.

p. 94, "You can't do everything": Berenice Kleiman, *Lessons Learned: Stroke Recovery from a Caregiver's Perspective* (Cleveland, OH: Cleveland Clinic Press, 2007): 28.

p. 95, Comments on asking for help: Gary Barg, editor, *The Fearless Caregiver: How to Get the Best Care for Your Loved One and Still Have a Life of Your Own* (Sterling, VA: Capitol Books, 2003).

p. 95, Caregiving as a "dance": Marty Richards, *Caresharing* (Woodstock, VT: Skylight Paths, 2009), 2.

p. 99, "A therapist is an emotion doctor": Dana Reeve, interview, in *The Fearless Caregiver,* edited by Gary Barg, 158.

p. 104, Guidelines for scheduling caregiver breaks: Gary Barg, editor, *The Fearless Caregiver,* 173 (our italics).

p. 110, "A Caregiver's Bill of Rights": This document, widely available on the Internet, has been adapted from *CareGiving: Helping an Aging Loved One,* by Jo Horne (Washington, DC: AARP Books, 1985).

p. 111, "I don't look at myself as a caregiver": Sandy Senor, "Tips from a Caregiver Husband," in *The Fearless Caregiver,* edited by Gary Barg, 73–77.

Chapter 5. In Sickness and in Health

p. 117, Not "his" problem, but "their" problem: John S. Rolland, *Families, Illness, and Disability* (New York: Basic Books, 1994), 241.

Epilogue

p. 177, Structured psychotherapy focused on coping with illness: Irene Pollin and Susan Baird Kanaan, *Medical Crisis Counseling: Short-Term Therapy for Long-Term Illness* (New York: W. W. Norton, 1995).

p. 178, Four characteristics of effective interventions: Steven Zarit and Elia Femia, "Behavioral and Psychosocial Interventions for Family Caregivers," *American Journal of Nursing* 108, no. 9 (2008) Supplement, 47–53.

p. 178, NYU Caregiver Intervention: This program was developed by Mary Mittelman at the New York University School of Medicine and has been implemented in community settings.

p. 179, Guided Care caregiver intervention: Jennifer Wolff, Erin Rand-Giovanetti, Sara Palmer, Stephen Wegener, Lisa Reider, Katherine Frey, et al., "Caregiving and Chronic Care: The Guided Care Program for Families and Friends," *Journal of Gerontology Medical Sciences* 64 (2009): 785–91. More information on Guided Care is available at www.guidedcare.org.

p. 179, Caregiving for You, Caregiving for Me: Rosalynn Carter Institute for Caregiving, www.rci.gsw.edu.

p. 179, Coping with Caregiving: This program was developed by Dolores Gallagher-Thompson and her colleagues at Stanford University School of Medicine and the Veterans Administration Palo Alto Healthcare System.

p. 180, Caregiving intervention by videoconferencing: Denise M. Taylor, Jill I. Cameron, Leenah Walsh, Sara McEwen, Aura Kagan, David L. Streiner, and Maria P. Huijbregts, "Exploring the Feasibility of Video-conference Delivery of a Self-Management Program to Rural Participants with Stroke," *Telemedicine Journal and e-Health* 15, no. 7 (September 2009): 646–54.

p. 181, Presidential Task Force on Caregivers: *Aging Issues Newsletter,* vol. VV, Special Convention Issue, July–August 2009, published by the APA Office on Aging; available online at www.apa.org/pi/aging/resources/newsletter/2009/07/issue.pdf.

Resources

Caregiving, Including Respite Care, Home Care, and Adult Day Care

Barg, Gary, ed. *The Fearless Caregiver: How to Get the Best Care for Your Loved One and Still Have a Life of Your Own.* Sterling, VA: Capital Books, 2001.

Caring Today Magazine, 34 Sherman Ct., Fairfield, CT 06824, 203-254-0783, www.caringtoday.com.

Kleiman, Berenice. *Lessons Learned: Stroke Recovery from a Caregiver's Perspective.* Cleveland, OH: Cleveland Clinic Press, 2007.

Mace, Nancy L., and Peter V. Rabins. *The 36-Hour Day: A Family Guide to Caring for Persons with Alzheimer Disease, Related Dementing Illnesses, and Memory Loss in Later Life.* 4th ed. New York: Wellness Central, 2007.

Meyer, Maria, and Paula Derr. *The Comfort of Home for Stroke: A Guide for Caregivers.* Portland, OR: CareTrust, 2007.

Strong, Maggie. *Mainstay: For the Well Spouse of the Chronically Ill: A Moving Personal Account and a Companion Guide.* Boston, MA: Little, Brown, 1988.

Today's Caregiver, a magazine of the Caregiver Media Group, 3350 Griffin Rd., Fort Lauderdale, FL 33312, www.caregiver.com.

AARP
601 E Street NW
Washington, DC 20049
202-434-2277
www.aarp.org
Provides information on hiring home care workers and choosing home health agencies.

Administration on Aging
1 Massachusetts Avenue NW
Washington, DC 20001
202-619-0724
www.aoa.gov

Alzheimer's Association
225 N. Michigan Avenue, Floor 17
Chicago, IL 60601
703-218-2477
www.alz.org

Eldercare Locator
Department of Health and Human Services
1-800-677-1116
www.eldercare.gov

Family Caregiver Alliance
180 Montgomery Street, Suite 1100
San Francisco, CA 94104
1-800-445-8106
www.caregiver.org

Family Caregiving 101
www.familycaregiving101.org

National Alliance for Caregiving
4720 Montgomery Lane, 5th floor
Bethesda, MD 20814
www.caregiving.org

National Family Caregivers Association
10605 Concord Street, Suite 501
Kensington, MD 20895-2504
1-800-896-3650
www.thefamilycaregiver.org

National Respite Care Locator
Chapel Hill Training-Outreach Project, Inc.
800 Eastowne Drive, Suite 105
Chapel Hill, NC 27514
919-490-5577
www.respitelocator.org/searchStates.asp

Rosalynn Carter Institute for Caregiving
Georgia Southwestern University
800 GSW Drive
Americus, GA 31709
229-928-1234
www.rci.gsw.edu
Promotes research, education, training, and advocacy
for caregiver issues.

Wellspouse Association
62 West Main Street, Suite H
Freehold, NJ 07728
1-800-838-0879
www.wellspouse.org

General Stroke Information

Caplan, Louis R. *Stroke.* New York: Demos Medical, 2006.

Marler, John R. *Stroke for Dummies.* Hoboken, NJ: Wiley, 2005.

National Institute of Neurological Disorders and Stroke. *Know Stroke: Know the Signs: Act in Time.* http://stroke.nih.gov/. Offers a wide range of materials about stroke prevention, treatment, and rehabilitation, from National Institutes of Health experts on stroke.

National Stroke Association. *Hope: The Stroke Recovery Guide.* www.stroke.org.

Rao, Paul R., Mark N. Ozer, and John E. Toerge, eds. *Managing Stroke: A Guide to Living Well after Stroke.* Washington, DC: NRH Press, 2000.

Senelick, Richard, and Karla Dougherty. *Living with Stroke: A Guide for Families.* Birmingham, AL: Health South Press, 2001.

Stein, Joel. *Stroke and the Family: A New Guide.* Cambridge, MA: Harvard University Press, 2004.

Stein, Joel, Julie Silver, and Elizabeth Pegg Frates. *Life after Stroke: The Guide to Recovering Your Health and Preventing Another Stroke.* Baltimore, MD: Johns Hopkins University Press, 2006.

Stroke Connection, a magazine of the American Stroke Association, www.strokeassociation.org.

Stroke Smart, a magazine of the National Stroke Association, www.stroke.org.

American Heart Association / American Stroke
Association
7272 Greenville Avenue
Dallas, TX 75231
1-800-242-8721
www.strokeassociation.org

Heart and Stroke Association of Canada
www.heartandstroke.ca

National Stroke Association
9707 East Easter Lane, Building B
Englewood, CO 80112
1-800-787-6537
www.stroke.org

Healthy Lifestyles

The New American Heart Association Cookbook. 7th ed. New York: Clarkson N.
Potter, 2007.

American Diabetes Association
Attn: National Call Center
1701 North Beauregard Street
Alexandria, VA 22311
1-800-DIABETES
www.diabetes.org
Information, education, and support for people with
diabetes; addresses nutrition, exercise, weight loss, and
prevention of complications.

HealthierUS.gov
www.healthierus.gov
U.S. government site promoting healthy living through
diet, exercise, smoking cessation, and more.

Smokefree.gov
www.smokefree.gov
U.S. government site providing information, support,
and resources to help people stop smoking.

Insurance

Mercer's 2010 Guide to Social Security. 38th ed. Louisville, KY: Mercer, 2010. Available online from www.mercer.com.

Mercer's 2010 Medicare Booklet. 27th ed. Louisville, KY: Mercer, 2010. Available online from www.mercer.com.

A Shoppers Guide to Long Term Care Insurance. Pamphlet published by the National Association of Insurance Commissioners, 120 W. Twelfth Street, Suite 100, Kansas City, MO 64105, 816-842-3600. Available online from www.naic.org.

Centers for Medicare and Medicaid Services (CMS)
U.S. Department of Health and Human Services
www.cms.hhs.gov
Information on Medicare and Medicaid benefits and programs, the Medicaid Waiver, and other programs and services provided by these government health insurance programs.

Medicare
1-800-MEDICARE
www.medicare.gov

Social Security Administration
www.ssa.gov
Information on Social Security disability and retirement benefits, the application process, and locating your local Social Security office.

U.S. Department of Veterans Affairs
Federal Benefits for Veterans, Dependents, and Survivors
www.va.gov/

Long-Term-Care Planning

Guide to Choosing a Nursing Home. Pamphlet published by the U.S. Government. Available free online at www.medicare.gov/Publications/Pubs/pdf/02174.pdf.

Certified Financial Planner Board of Standards
1425 K Street NW, Suite 500
Washington, DC 20005
1-800-487-1497
www.cfp.net
This is the board that certifies financial planners. The
Web site provides a locator service you can use to find
a Certified Financial Planner in your local area.

ElderLawAnswers
260 West Exchange Street, Suite 004
Box 29
Providence, RI 02903
1-866-267-0947
www.elderlawanswers.com
Information on long-term care, insurance, advance
directives; a list of elder-care lawyers by location.

National Clearinghouse for Long Term Care
Information
U.S. Department of Health and Human Services
www.longtermcare.gov

Memoirs

Bauby, Jean-Dominique. *The Diving Bell and the Butterfly.* New York: Vintage
Books, 1997.
Garrison, Julia Fox. *Don't Leave Me Like This: Or When I Get Back on My Feet
You'll Be Sorry.* New York: HarperCollins, 2006.
Kassel, Pat, ed. *The Best of the Stroke Connection: A Collection of Personal Stories
by Stroke Survivors and Caregivers.* Golden Valley, MN: Courage Press, 1990.
Kleiman, Berenice, and Herb Kleiman. *One Stroke, Two Survivors: The Incredi-
ble Journey of Berenice and Herb Kleiman.* Cleveland, OH: Cleveland Clinic
Press, 2006.
McCrum, Robert. *My Year Off: Recovering Life after Stroke.* New York: W. W.
Norton, 1998.
McEwan, Mark. *Change in the Weather: Life after Stroke.* New York: Gotham
Books, 2008.
Taylor, Jill Bolte. *My Stroke of Insight: A Brain Scientist's Personal Journey.* New
York: Viking, 2006.

Mental Health and Couples Therapy

"Caregiver Assessment Tool." www.ama-assn.org/ama/upload/mm/36/care givertooleng.pdf. A short quiz that can give you an idea of your stress level and whether you should consider seeking treatment from a doctor or getting more support. Includes phone numbers for caregiver organizations. Created by the American Medical Association.

American Association of Marriage and Family
Therapists
112 South Alfred Street
Alexandria, VA 22314-3061
703-838-9808
Provides a Therapist Locator service (www.therapist locator.net) to help you find a qualified marriage therapist in your local area.

American Psychiatric Association
1000 Wilson Boulevard, Suite 1825
Arlington, VA 22209
1-800-35-PSYCH
www.psych.org

American Psychological Association
750 First Street NE
Washington, DC 20002
1-800-374-2721
www.apa.org

National Association of Social Workers
750 First Street NE, Suite 700
Washington, DC 20002
202-408-8600
www.socialworkers.org

National Institute of Mental Health
Science Writing, Press, and Dissemination Branch
6001 Executive Boulevard, Room 8184, MSC 9663
Bethesda, MD 20892-9663
1-866-615-6464
www.nimh.nih.gov

Recreation, Sports, and Travel

Access-Able Travel Source
P.O. Box 1796
Wheat Ridge, CO 80034
www.access-able.com

Disabled Sports USA
451 Hungerford Drive, Suite 100
Rockville, MD 20850
301-217-0960
www.dsusa.org
Promotes sports for people with disabilities.

Disabled Travel Agency Directory
www.dmoz.org/Society/Disabled/Travel/Agencies
A directory of travel agencies with services for people
with disabilities.

National Sports Center for the Disabled
P.O. Box 1290
Winter Park, CO 80482
970-726-1540
www.nscd.org
Offers summer and winter sports and recreation
programs for people with disabilities.

Retreat & Refresh Stroke Camp
425 W. Giles Lane
Peoria, IL 61614
1-866-688-5450
www.strokecamp.org
Offers weekend camping for stroke survivors and their
family caregivers.

United States Adaptive Golf Association
P.O. Box 708
Far Hills, NJ 07931
908-234-2300

www.usaga.org
Promotes golf for persons with disabilities.

U.S. Adaptive Recreation Center
P.O. Box 2897, 43101 Goldmine Drive
Big Bear Lake, CA 92315
909-584-0269 (voice); 1-800-735-2929 (TTY)
www.usarc.org
Sponsors adaptive skiing, water sports, and camping
for people with disabilities.

Sexuality

American Heart Association. *Sex after Stroke: Our Guide to Intimacy after Stroke.*
Pamphlet published in 2008 and distributed by Krames. Order by phone
(1-800-333-3032) or online (www.krames.com/aha).

Caswell, John. "Sex and Intimacy after Stroke." *Stroke Connection,* March–
April 2009.

National Stroke Association. *Recovery after Stroke: Redefining Sexuality.* Fact
Sheet published by the NSA Publications Committee, National Stroke
Association, 2006. Order by phone (1-800-787-6537) or obtain free online
(www.stroke.org).

American Association of Sexuality Educators,
Counselors, and Therapists
P.O. Box 1960
Ashland, VA 23005-1960
804-752-0026
www.aasect.org

Sexual Health Network
www.sexualhealth.com
Information about sexuality, including "Disability and
Chronic Conditions."

Speech-Language and Swallowing Disorders

APHASIA

National Institute on Deafness and other Communicative Disorders.
Aphasia. www.nidcd.nih.gov/health/voice/aphasia.asp. Offers a range of

information about aphasia, including links to other sites, from NIH experts on aphasia.

American Speech-Language-Hearing Association
10801 Rockville Pike
Rockville, MD 20852
1-800-498-2071 (voice); 301-897-5700 (TTY)

National Aphasia Association
156 Fifth Avenue, Suite 707
New York, NY 10010
1-800-922-4622
www.aphasia.org
An organization for people with aphasia and their families.

DYSPHAGIA (SWALLOWING DISORDERS)

National Institute on Deafness and other Communicative Disorders, *Dysphagia.* www.nidcd.nih.gov/health/voice/dysph.asp. Offers a range of information about dysphagia, including links to other sites, from NIH experts on swallowing disorders.

Wilson, J. Randy *I-Can't-Chew Cookbook: Delicious Soft Diet Recipes for People with Chewing, Swallowing, and Dry Mouth Disorders.* Alameda, CA: Hunter House, 2003.

Index